The

TAKE
CARE of
YOURSELF
GUIDE

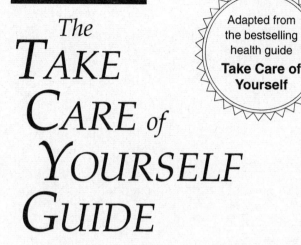

Adapted from
the bestselling
health guide
**Take Care of
Yourself**

TO TREATING YOUR FAMILY'S MOST COMMON SYMPTOMS

Donald M. Vickery, M.D.
James F. Fries, M.D.

PERSEUS BOOKS
Reading, Massachusetts

Perseus Books are available at special discounts for bulk purchases in the U.S. by corporations, institutions, and other organizations. For more information, please contact the Special Markets Department at HarperCollins Publishers, 10 East 53rd Street, New York, NY 10022, or call 212-207-7528.

0-7382-0062-X

Perseus Books is a member of the Perseus Books Group

Abridged by Bruce Goldfarb from the sixth edition of *Take Care of Yourself*
Edited by John Bell
Cover design © 1998 by Mike Stromberg

Set in 10-point Palatino by Eclipse Publishing Services, Nashua, N.H.

1 2 3 4 5 6 7 8 9-DOC-030201009998
First printing, June 1998

INTRODUCTION

You can do more for your health than your doctor can.

We introduced our book *Take Care of Yourself* with that phrase in 1976. Then as now, our society depended too heavily on medical experts of every kind, and on complex gadgetry and medications. But today the idea that your health depends largely on *you*—the *Take Care of Yourself* strategy—is nationally accepted.

There have been more than a hundred printings of *Take Care of Yourself*, totaling more than 11 million copies. It has been the central feature of many programs sponsored by corporations, health insurance plans, and other institutions to promote health. We're proud that our book played a role in changing the perception of good health care.

Does the *Take Care of Yourself* approach work? Can a book help you to improve your health? Can you learn to stay healthy while using your doctor and other medical resources less and reducing your out-of-pocket costs? Absolutely. *Take Care of Yourself* has received extensive scientific evaluation, with results published in peer-reviewed medical journals such as the *Journal of the American Medical Association*. Five major scientific studies show that the book can reduce medical visits and health care costs.

Now we have put the most useful advice in *Take Care of Yourself* into this shorter guide. We have tried to make this book easy for you to read and refer to, so that more people can enjoy the benefits of the *Take Care of Yourself* approach.

Why should you work to reduce health care costs when you have insurance to pay them? It's important to understand that every procedure performed on every patient adds to the total health care bill we share.

Furthermore, by avoiding unneeded medical care you'll have more time for yourself, and you'll reduce your exposure to medical tests, medication side effects, and other unavoidable risks in health care. Overall, you're better off if your care is simple and under your control.

Most important, good health is its own reward. A vigorous lifestyle, a sense of adventure and excitement, and the ability to make choices and take responsibility for yourself are essential to—and benefits of—the healthy life. Take care of yourself. Your loved ones will thank you for it.

CAUTIONS

This book's medical advice is sound and reasonable, but it will not always work. Everybody responds differently to illness and injury. We wanted to make the book as specific and detailed as possible. In doing so, we may give information and advice that are just not right for you. Use reasonable judgment when considering information in this guide. It is a supplement to your health care, not a substitute for it. Specifically, do the following:

- If you're under a doctor's care, listen to your doctor and not this book. This is especially important if you have been diagnosed with a chronic health condition.
- Read medicine label directions carefully.
- Check with a health care professional if you may be allergic to a medication recommended in this book.
- Call your health care provider if the problem persists longer than reasonable.

CONTENTS

HOW TO USE THIS GUIDE

We've tried to make this book very easy for you to use. We want you to be able to quickly find the information you need, from emergency care, to responses to specific symptoms, to preventive measures that will help you stay healthy.

Follow these steps if you have a medical problem:

1. **Determine whether it is an emergency.** Read pages 4–5 *now* to learn about emergencies. Learning what to do will prepare you before a crisis strikes. Usually emergencies are obvious. Fortunately, they are rare.

2. **Look up your chief complaint or symptom.** The table of contents lists the most common medical symptoms, organized by type. You can also look up symptoms in the index. If you have more than one symptom—such as abdominal pain, nausea, *and* diarrhea—look up the most severe problem first.

3. **Read the general information in that section.** Each section describes:

   - a problem
   - its likely causes, signs, and symptoms
   - how to treat it at home
   - what to expect at a doctor's office

4. **Go through the decision chart.** Each section has a decision chart to guide your care, like the example shown on page 2. Start at the top of the chart. Answer every question and follow the arrows suggested by your answers. If a box asks a series of questions, and you can answer yes to any of them, follow the yes arrow. The decision chart will help

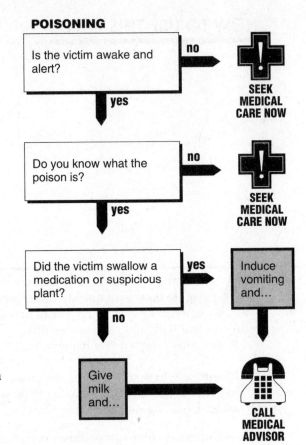

POISONING

Is the victim awake and alert?

no → **SEEK MEDICAL CARE NOW**

yes ↓

Do you know what the poison is?

no → **SEEK MEDICAL CARE NOW**

yes ↓

Did the victim swallow a medication or suspicious plant?

yes → Induce vomiting and...

no ↓

Give milk and... → **CALL MEDICAL ADVISOR**

Sample decision chart. Each symptom section has a chart. Start at the top question, and follow the arrows suggested by your answers.

you decide whether you need a doctor's attention or can use home treatment. If you use more than one chart, play it safe. If one chart suggests home treatment and another advises calling the doctor, call the doctor. Better to err on the side of caution.

5. **Follow the advice suggested by the decision chart.** The decision charts recommend one of the following actions:

- **Seek Medical Care Now.** You need prompt medical attention. Arrange to see your doctor or go to a medical facility.

- **Seek Medical Care Today.**   Call your doctor's office or health line and describe your condition over the phone as clearly as you can. Most likely, a doctor will want to see you right away.

- **Make Medical Appointment.**   Schedule a visit with your doctor or health care professional at the earliest opportunity, ideally within a few days.

- **Call Medical Advisor.**   A talk over the phone with a doctor or nurse may resolve your health issue without the need for an office visit. Few doctors charge for telephone advice for regular patients, so long as you do not call much more often than you need to. Many health plans have phone advice lines set up for you.

- **Use Home Treatment.**   Follow the directions for home treatment. Using home treatment doesn't mean your condition is trivial. The home treatments in this book are steps doctors often recommend during an office visit. Call or see your doctor if a good trial of home treatment fails to take care of your problem.

6. **At your leisure, read the last three sections of the book.**   "Preventing Health Problems" will help you lead a healthier life, and a longer one. "Working with Your Health Care Team" explains how to get the most out of your relationship with doctors, nurses, and pharmacists. And "Your Home Pharmacy" tells exactly what you should keep in your house for everyday medical problems or emergencies.

EMERGENCIES

If a person has a condition that may pose a risk to life or limb, you must get help immediately. Depending on the person's condition and your situation, the quickest way may be to:

- Drive the victim to the hospital emergency department. Have someone call ahead.
- Call the 911 emergency number. Many communities are served by emergency medical services (EMS). Trained crews sent to your home can begin treatment before a person arrives at the hospital.
- Call the local poison information center or emergency departments. For poisoning, these sources can often tell you how to begin treatment as early as possible.

EMERGENCY SIGNS

Emergency signs are signals that a person needs immediate medical attention. Familiarity with emergency signs will enable you to do the right thing at the right time, and to provide reassurance when a condition is not life-threatening.

The decision charts presented in this book assume that the problems are not emergencies. If you see any of these emergency signs, seek immediate medical attention:

No Pulse or Breath

The absence of a heartbeat or breathing is a life-threatening emergency. Call for help. If you know cardiopulmonary resuscitation (CPR), begin rescue breathing or chest compressions as needed. See page 6 to read about choking.

The best way to learn CPR and first aid is through hands-on instruction provided by your local American Red Cross, American Heart Association, or a nearby hospital or college. We urge you to take these classes.

Major Injury

Major injuries need immediate medical attention. While hard to define, a major injury is one that involves more than one body system (muscle, bone, blood vessels, nerves, etc.), or one that could be disabling. Such injuries include the fracture of a leg or other large bone, or possible injury to the head or back. Trauma to the chest and abdomen are often major injuries. Usually a major injury is obvious.

Bleeding

Bleeding can be dramatic but often makes an injury look a lot worse than it really is. The average adult can tolerate the loss of several cups of blood with little ill effect. Losing blood is more dangerous for children because of their smaller size. Applying pressure directly on a wound, preferably with a sterile dressing, can stop most bleeding. If you can't control the bleeding by direct pressure, the person requires immediate medical attention.

Unconsciousness or Stupor

A person who is unconscious and can't be roused needs immediate emergency care. "Stupor" is a decreased level of mental activity while the person is still conscious. A drowsy or stuporous person who cannot respond to questioning or gentle shaking should also receive urgent attention. Judging changes of consciousness in children can be difficult. Treat as an emergency a child whom you cannot rouse.

Disorientation

Head injury, fever, and other medical conditions can cause confusion and disorientation. Doctors assess disorientation of *time, place,* and *person*—the patient's ability to correctly answer these questions:

- What is today's date?
- Where are we?
- Who are you?

A previously alert person who becomes disoriented or confused requires immediate medical attention.

Shortness of Breath

As a rule, a person who is short of breath or has difficulty breathing while at rest should receive immediate medical attention. We discuss shortness of breath in more detail on page 86. If you aren't sure about the cause and proper care of shortness of breath, you should seek aid immediately.

Sweating

As an isolated sign, sweating isn't usually serious. It is a normal response to elevated temperature and to psychological or physical stress. Aspirin can cause sweating when lowering a fever. A "cold sweat," however, is a common sign of severe pain, serious illness, or injury. The person in a cold sweat may have skin that is pale, cool, and clammy. A cold sweat in a person with chest pain, abdominal pain, or light-headedness suggests the need for immediate medical attention.

Severe Pain

Pain is one of the most common reasons people seek emergency care. By itself, pain does not indicate the seriousness or urgency of a problem. A minor injury may be quite painful, while a very serious medical condition can cause little or no pain. Most often, pain is associated with other signs or symptoms that suggest the urgency of a condition, such as shortness of breath or sweating. Severe pain demands urgent medical attention, if for no other reason than pain relief.

AMBULANCES

Not all urgent problems require the top level of emergency response. If it is practical and does not cause discomfort to the patient, it may be quicker to drive the person to the emergency department in your own car than to wait for an ambulance to come to your home. In general, call an ambulance for a person who:

- Is gravely ill
- May have an injury to the head or back
- May be suffering a heart attack
- Is severely short of breath
- Cannot be transported to the hospital by car

CHOKING

Choking is a life-threatening emergency that requires your immediate attention. Food or a foreign object can partially or completely block a person's airway, obstructing the flow of air to the lungs. Emergency services play virtually no role in helping a choking victim; actions by the people at the scene determine whether he or she will survive.

The most common cause of choking in adults is food, often a solid meat such as steak. The victim is likely to have been drinking alcoholic beverages, which slow the reflexes that keep food from going down the wrong way. Often, talking or laughing has distracted the victim from eating safely.

Children put a variety of objects into their mouths and do so at any time of day or night. Even so, the most common cause of choking in children is food—hot dogs, grapes, peanuts, and hard candy.

Recognizing the signs of choking is important. The choking person:

- Cannot speak, cough, or cry out
- Cannot breathe, and may turn blue
- May, if he or she has learned this emergency sign, put one hand to the throat

HOME TREATMENT

Your prompt action can make the difference between life and death for the choking victim. Once you determine that the person is choking, the most effective way to unblock the airway is with the abdominal thrust, or Heimlich maneuver (below). Compressing the lungs creates air pressure behind the foreign object, forcing it out of the airway.

Done properly, abdominal thrusts do not pose a great risk of harm to the victim. Still, you should not do the maneuver needlessly on a person who is not choking. A person who is coughing violently is not choking.

Adult Victim

1. Stand behind the choking victim and place your arms around him or her.

2. Make a fist and place it against the victim's abdomen, thumb side in, between the navel and the ribs.

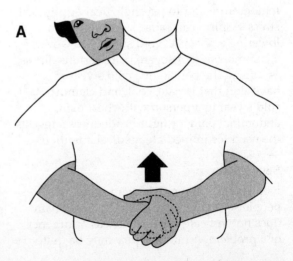

A

Abdominal thrust (Heimlich maneuver) for standing adults.

CHOKING

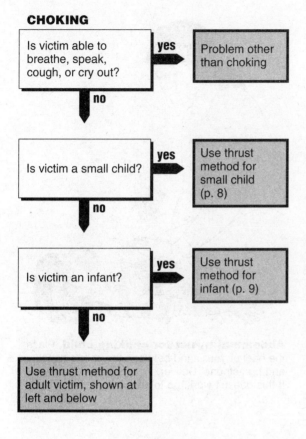

| Is victim able to breathe, speak, cough, or cry out? | **yes** → | Problem other than choking |

↓ **no**

| Is victim a small child? | **yes** → | Use thrust method for small child (p. 8) |

↓ **no**

| Is victim an infant? | **yes** → | Use thrust method for infant (p. 9) |

↓ **no**

| Use thrust method for adult victim, shown at left and below |

3. Hold the fist with your other hand. Give four quick thrusts upward and inward with your fists.

If the victim is pregnant or obese, place your arms around his or her chest and your hands over the middle of the breastbone. Give four quick chest thrusts.

If the victim is lying down, roll the victim onto his or her back. Place your hands on the abdomen between the navel and the ribs and push upward and inward (below). Give four quick abdominal thrusts.

If the victim is much taller or heavier than you, have the victim lie on the floor and use the lying-down method described above.

4. If the victim *still* isn't breathing, lift the jaw and tongue and look for the object causing the obstruction. *If you can see the object,* sweep it out of the mouth with your finger. If you try to remove an object you can't see, you may push it further into the airway.

5. If the victim *still* isn't breathing after the object is removed, begin mouth-to-mouth rescue breathing.

6. Call for help, and repeat these steps until the object is removed and the victim is breathing normally.

B

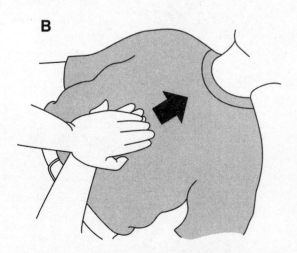

Abdominal thrust (Heimlich maneuver) for adults lying down.

For Choking Child

1. Have the child lie down. Kneel at victim's side.

2. Position the heel of one hand on the child's abdomen between the navel and the breastbone.

3. Deliver six to ten inward and upward thrusts.

4. If the child *still* isn't breathing, lift the jaw and tongue and look inside the mouth for the object obstructing the airway. *If you can see the object*, sweep it out of the throat with your finger. Trying to remove an object that you can't see may push it further into the airway.

5. If the child *still* isn't breathing after you have removed the object, begin mouth-to-mouth rescue breathing.

6. Call for help, and repeat these steps until you remove the object and the child is breathing normally again.

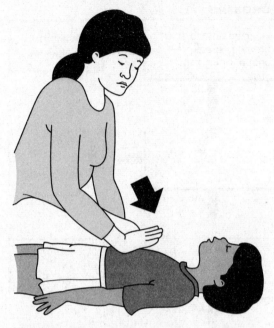

Abdominal thrust for choking child. Place the heel of your hand between the child's navel and breastbone. Deliver six to ten quick thrusts. If this doesn't work, go to step 4.

For Choking Infant

1. Hold the infant along your forearm, face forward, with the head lower than the feet.

2. Deliver four rapid blows to the back, between the shoulder blades, with the heel of your hand.

3. If the baby *still* isn't breathing, turn him or her over and, using two fingers, give four quick upward thrusts to the chest.

4. If the baby *still* isn't breathing, lift the tongue and jaw and look inside the mouth for the object causing the obstruction. *If you can see the object*, gently sweep it out with your little finger. Trying to remove an object you can't see may push it further into the airway.

5. If the baby *still* isn't breathing after you remove the object, give rescue breathing by mouth-to-mouth-and-nose.

6. Call for help, and repeat these steps until you remove the object and the baby is breathing normally.

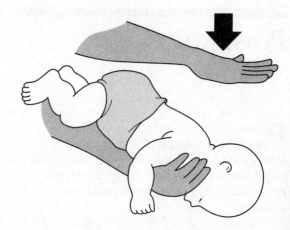

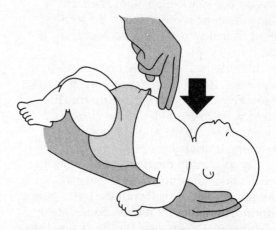

Abdominal thrust for choking infant. If four rapid blows to the infant's back don't work, deliver four quick thrusts to the infant's chest as shown above.

POISONING

Poisoning is one of the most common household emergencies, particularly among children. Although some poisons can be inhaled or absorbed through the skin, in most poisoning emergencies they are swallowed.

"Food poisoning" is a term sometimes used to describe digestive problems that don't have an obvious explanation. The care for food poisoning is described in the sections about Diarrhea (p. 90) and Nausea and Vomiting (p. 88).

Identifying a poisoning promptly is important. If you suspect a poisoning, don't panic. Few cases of poisoning are true life-threatening emergencies. If the victim is unconscious, call 911 and give rescue breathing if needed.

Try to identify the type of poison, if that doesn't take too much time. If you can identify the poison, call your doctor or poison information center for advice. Follow their recommendations to care for the victim. Bring along any containers and bottles to the hospital, along with material vomited by the victim.

A drug overdose could be a suicide attempt. Someone who has attempted suicide with poison needs help, first to recover from the overdose and then to overcome his or her self-destructive feelings.

HOME TREATMENT

All cases of poisoning require medical help. By consulting with a doctor or poison informa-tion center, however, people can manage many cases of poisoning at home with careful observation of the victim.

If the victim is conscious and the poison is known, the doctor or poison information center will advise you whether or not to induce vomiting. Vomiting should *not* be induced if the victim has swallowed any of the following:

- Acids: battery acid, sulfuric acid, hydro-chloric acid, bleach, hair straighteners, etc.
- Alkalis: Drano and other drain cleaners, oven cleaners, etc.
- Petroleum products: gasoline, furniture polish, kerosene, lighter fluid, etc.

These substances can damage the esophagus and lungs if vomited. Neutralize them with milk, water, or milk of magnesia while calling for help.

For other poisons, vomiting is a safe way to remove them from the stomach. One of the fastest ways to induce vomiting is to touch the back of the victim's throat with a finger. Collect the vomited material and take it to be examined by the doctor.

You can also induce vomiting with 2 to 4 teaspoons (10 to 20 ml) of syrup of ipecac, followed by as much liquid as the victim can drink. Vomiting usually follows within 20 minutes. Mustard mixed in warm water also works. Repeat the dose if vomiting does not result within 25 minutes.

Once the crisis of poisoning has passed, take steps to make sure it doesn't happen again. Put poisons out of a child's reach.

WHAT TO EXPECT

Severe cases of poisoning are best managed in the hospital emergency department, not the doctor's office. Treatment depends on the type

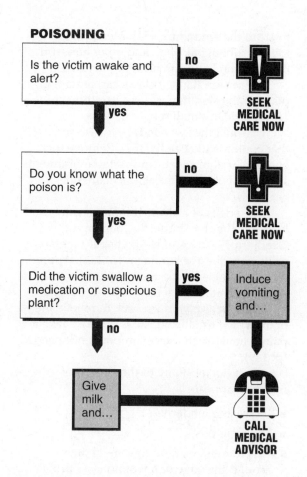

POISONING

Is the victim awake and alert?

no → **SEEK MEDICAL CARE NOW**

yes ↓

Do you know what the poison is?

no → **SEEK MEDICAL CARE NOW**

yes ↓

Did the victim swallow a medication or suspicious plant?

yes → Induce vomiting and…

no ↓

Give milk and… → **CALL MEDICAL ADVISOR**

PREVENTING POISONINGS

Most cases of poisoning can be prevented. Children almost always swallow poison unintentionally. Keep potentially harmful substances out of their reach:

- Store harmful substances in their original, labeled containers in a secure area.
- Don't give children access to medications, insecticides, caustic cleaners, solvents, fuels, furniture polish, antifreeze, and drain cleaners.
- Keep drugs in child-resistant containers. Flush old medicines down the toilet.

of poison, the amount remaining in the body, and the victim's health status. The victim's stomach may be emptied by vomiting or use of a stomach pump. The staff may give the victim activated charcoal to absorb poison from the digestive tract. Victims who are unconscious or have swallowed a caustic substance may be admitted to the hospital for longer observation and treatment.

CUTS AND SCRAPES

You can care for most common skin injuries and minor wounds in your home.

Scrapes and abrasions are shallow wounds of the skin. They may tear or scrape off top layers of the skin, but the wound does not affect deeper skin layers or underlying tissue. Because scrapes injure many nerve endings at once, they're usually more painful than cuts.

Most cuts affect only the skin and superficial tissue and heal without lasting effects. Deeper wounds involving blood vessels, nerves, tendons, ligaments, and other underlying tissues can cause permanent damage.

Signs that a cut needs a doctor's attention include:

- Bleeding that you can't control with pressure—an **emergency** (p. 4).
- Numbness or weakness in the limb beyond the wound
- Inability to move the fingers or toes
- Signs of infection: pus, fever, extensive redness and swelling after 24 hours or more
- Cuts to the chest, abdomen, or back, unless they are very small or shallow

HOME TREATMENT

Stop the bleeding by pressing directly on the wound, using a sterile dressing if available. Remove dirt and foreign matter from the wound, and vigorously wash the area with soap and water. Make sure no debris remains inside. You can use 3% hydrogen peroxide or an antiseptic such as Betadine or Merthiolate to clean the wound (p. 154). Mercurochrome, iodine, rubbing alcohol, and other antiseptics do little good and can be very painful.

Loose skin flaps, if clean, can remain in place. If the skin flap is dirty, carefully cut it off with clean, small scissors.

Use an adhesive bandage for wounds that continue to ooze (p. 154). Remove the bandage if it gets wet. Antibacterial ointments such as Neosporin or Bacitracin are not necessary.

The edges of a clean, minor cut can be held together by "butterfly" bandages, "steristrips" (strips of sterile paper tape), or ordinary adhesive bandages (p. 154). Apply these bandages so the wound edges join without "rolling under."

You can apply an ice pack to relieve the pain, which usually subsides quickly. Take a pain reliever such as acetaminophen if needed (p. 149).

See a doctor if any of these signs of infection appear:

- Increasing tenderness
- Draining pus
- Severe redness, though some redness around the edge of a wound is a normal part of healing

See a doctor if the wound isn't healing well after two weeks.

WHAT TO EXPECT

The doctor will clean the wound of dirt and foreign matter and assess the extent of injury to skin and underlying tissues.

The doctor may use a local anesthetic, such as Xylocaine, to numb the area around the wound. Tell the doctor if you are allergic to anesthetics. The doctor may also give a tetanus shot and antibiotics. The doctor may

CUTS AND SCRAPES

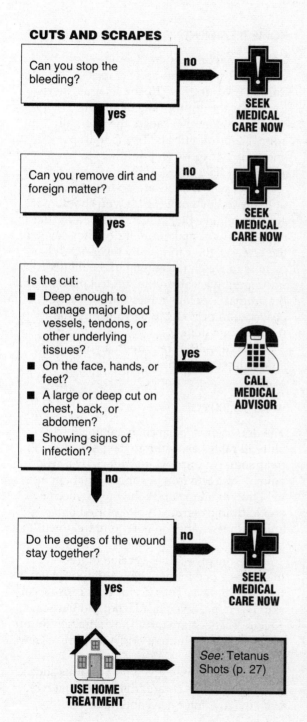

Can you stop the bleeding? — **no** → **SEEK MEDICAL CARE NOW**

yes ↓

Can you remove dirt and foreign matter? — **no** → **SEEK MEDICAL CARE NOW**

yes ↓

Is the cut:
- Deep enough to damage major blood vessels, tendons, or other underlying tissues?
- On the face, hands, or feet?
- A large or deep cut on chest, back, or abdomen?
- Showing signs of infection?

yes → **CALL MEDICAL ADVISOR**

no ↓

Do the edges of the wound stay together? — **no** → **SEEK MEDICAL CARE NOW**

yes ↓

USE HOME TREATMENT → *See:* Tetanus Shots (p. 27)

apply antibiotic ointment and a sterile dressing over the wound to promote healing.

A surgical specialist may tend to injuries to tendons or major blood vessels, especially those of the hands or face.

STITCHES

Stitches keep the edges of a cut together, helping it to heal and limiting scarring. Not all cuts require stitches. If the edges of a wound stay together, a sterile dressing or adhesive bandage is usually all you need.

Stitching should be done within eight hours of the injury. Otherwise a wound may not heal properly. In general, stitches may be required for:

- Cuts on the face
- Cuts on the hands or feet
- Cuts on the elbow, knee, or other area that bends often
- Cuts with edges that won't stay together
- Children who are likely to pull off bandages

Your doctor will tell you when the stitches should be removed. You can often do this at home with clean tweezers and a pair of small, sharp scissors:

1. Clean the skin and the stitches with soap and water. Soaking will help remove scabs.
2. With the tweezers, grasp a loose end of a knot and gently lift the stitch from the skin.
3. Cut the stitch as close to the skin as possible.
4. Lift the tweezers, pulling out the part of the stitch that had been under the skin.

ANIMAL BITES

Rabies is a very serious viral infection carried in the saliva of animals. It can be transmitted to humans through a bite or scratch. Although three thousand to four thousand animals with rabies are found in the United States each year, only one or two people get the disease.

A rabid animal may behave in strange ways:

- Not running from humans as you would expect
- Attacking without provocation
- Drooling or foaming at the mouth
- Walking around in the daytime if it is normally nocturnal

Avoid animals that act out of the ordinary.

The main carriers of rabies are skunks, foxes, bats, and raccoons. Rabies is less common in cattle, dogs, and cats. The disease is extremely rare in squirrels, chipmunks, rats, and mice. Cats and dogs pose the greatest risk of rabies to people because of their frequent contact with humans and the large number of bites reported each year. For the sake of your pets, your neighbors, and yourself, immunize your cats and dogs against rabies.

If you have been bitten by a wild animal, or by a dog or cat whose immunization history you don't know, call your doctor to decide whether you need antirabies treatment.

If you have been bitten by a pet dog or cat, and the animal's owner has its shots up to date and will observe the animal for sickness, you don't need to go to the doctor.

HOME TREATMENT

Treat animal bites as you would other wounds. Turn to Cuts and Scrapes (p. 12), Puncture Wounds (p. 16), or Tetanus Shots (p. 27) for the appropriate treatment.

If a wild animal causes the bite, call animal control officials. Trying to trap a wild animal may expose you or others to additional risk.

A pet whose shots are up to date is unlikely to have rabies. Still, you should arrange to have the animal observed for the next 15 days to make sure it does not develop the disease. You can usually rely on pet owners to watch the animal. If the owner is uncooperative, call animal control officials. If the animal develops rabies during the observation period, bite victims must be treated immediately.

Many localities require that you report animal bites to the health department.

WHAT TO EXPECT

The doctor must balance the remote possibility of rabies exposure to the risks of treatment. An unprovoked attack by a wild animal, or a bite from an animal that appears to be rabid, may require the rabies vaccine and antirabies serum. A bite caused by an animal that escaped may require treatment to be safe.

Doctors give rabies vaccine in five injections—one immediately and four over the next 28 days. The vaccine may cause local skin reactions, fever, headache, and nausea. Severe reactions are rare. The antirabies serum used today is of human origin and causes few side effects.

The doctor may give you a tetanus shot, although tetanus is rare from an animal bite. Usually you don't need antibiotics.

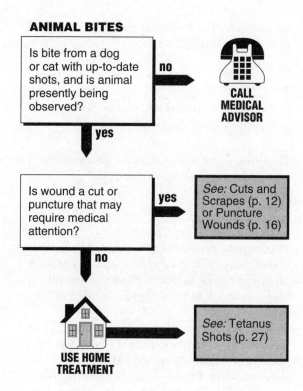

ANIMAL BITES

Is bite from a dog or cat with up-to-date shots, and is animal presently being observed?

no → **CALL MEDICAL ADVISOR**

yes ↓

Is wound a cut or puncture that may require medical attention?

yes → *See:* Cuts and Scrapes (p. 12) or Puncture Wounds (p. 16)

no ↓

USE HOME TREATMENT → *See:* Tetanus Shots (p. 27)

Puncture Wounds

Nails, pins, tacks, and other sharp objects can cause puncture wounds of the skin. Since puncture wounds rarely need stitches, the important questions are:

- Are the underlying tissues injured?
- Is anything (dirt or object) left in the wound?
- Does the victim need a tetanus shot?

Most minor puncture wounds involve the extremities—arms, hands, legs, and especially feet. A deep puncture elsewhere on the body could cause internal injury that is not obvious, so call the doctor for advice. A puncture wound on the hand can be serious if it gets infected. Call the doctor for a wound of the hand unless it is very minor.

A nail, ice pick, or other large object is more likely to cause underlying injury than a narrow item like a needle. The rare signs of serious injury are:

- Blood pumping vigorously from the wound—possible injured artery
- Numbness or tingling in the limb beyond the wound—possible injured nerves
- Difficulty moving the limb beyond the wound—possible injured tendon

These symptoms require **emergency** care.

Puncture wounds can become infected, especially if foreign material remains inside—a splinter, needle, or piece of glass. See the doctor if you have any question whether the wound is free of foreign material. Signs of infection include:

- Fever
- Extensive redness
- The formation of thick, yellowish pus
- Swelling of the area around the wound

These are signs to see a doctor and usually take 24 hours or more to develop.

HOME TREATMENT

Don't apply pressure to the wound unless it bleeds heavily or pumps in a way suggesting an artery has been injured. Let the wound bleed as much as possible to remove foreign material.

Clean the wound with soap and water or 3% hydrogen peroxide (p. 154). Soak the wound in warm water or a baking soda solution several times a day for four to five days (p. 154). This helps keep the skin puncture open so that germs or foreign debris can drain from it.

Seek medical care if you see signs of infection or if the wound hasn't healed after two weeks.

Make sure you are immunized against tetanus (p. 27).

WHAT TO EXPECT

The doctor will examine the wound to assess the extent of the puncture, injury to underlying tissues, and possible infection. He or she may have X-rays taken or explore the wound surgically. Be prepared to tell the doctor about possible allergies to local anesthetics, such as Xylocaine. Most doctors recommend home treatment. Antibiotics are rarely prescribed.

PUNCTURE WOUNDS

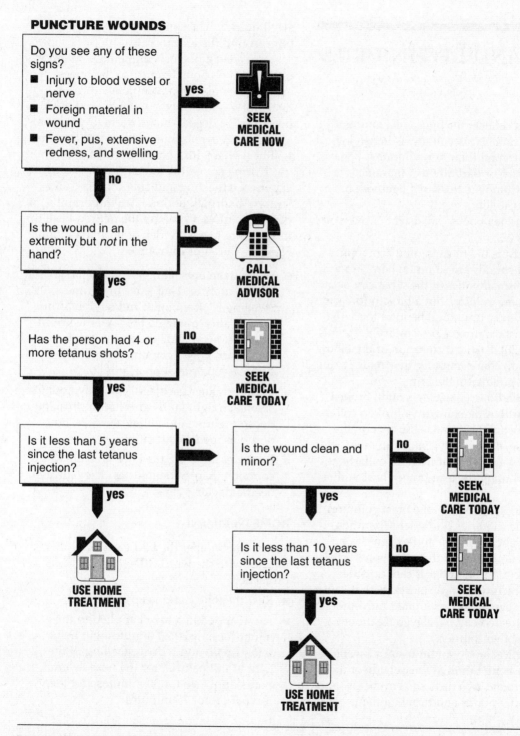

Do you see any of these signs?
- Injury to blood vessel or nerve
- Foreign material in wound
- Fever, pus, extensive redness, and swelling

yes → SEEK MEDICAL CARE NOW

no ↓

Is the wound in an extremity but *not* in the hand?

no → CALL MEDICAL ADVISOR

yes ↓

Has the person had 4 or more tetanus shots?

no → SEEK MEDICAL CARE TODAY

yes ↓

Is it less than 5 years since the last tetanus injection?

no → Is the wound clean and minor?

yes ↓

USE HOME TREATMENT

Is the wound clean and minor?

no → SEEK MEDICAL CARE TODAY

yes ↓

Is it less than 10 years since the last tetanus injection?

no → SEEK MEDICAL CARE TODAY

yes ↓

USE HOME TREATMENT

ARM AND LEG INJURIES

Ligaments connect the bones of a joint and provide stability as you move. When joints are forced beyond their normal limits, you can stretch (strain) or partially tear (sprain) ligaments. Complete tears of a ligament are rare outside athletics.

Arm and leg bones can also be broken or chipped (p. 22).

The wrist is the most injured arm joint. Strains and sprains are common here. Fractures of the small bones of the wrist can be hard to see on an X-ray, but a broken forearm puts an obvious, unnatural bend in the wrist.

The most common elbow injury is "tennis elbow" (p. 70). Partial dislocation of the elbow is common in children under five, usually due to an adult pulling on the arm.

The collarbone (clavicle) is often broken, but heals well. A person with a broken collarbone may be unable to raise the arm on the affected side, or may have shoulders that appear uneven. The treatment for collarbone injury is splinting the arm to the chest with a bandage.

Separation is perhaps the most common injury of the shoulder. Shoulder separation causes a slight deformity and extreme tenderness at the end of the collarbone. Actual dislocation of the shoulder is rare outside athletics. Fractures and dislocations that cause deformity, severe pain, or limited movement should be treated early. Delayed treatment won't hurt other injuries.

The typical ankle sprain usually swells around the bony bump at the outside of the ankle, or around two inches (5 cm) below and in front of it. Sprains and torn ligaments often swell quickly. The skin may turn black-and-blue around the affected area.

You need a doctor's immediate attention only for an obvious fracture to the bones around the ankle or a completely torn ligament. See the doctor if the injured ankle is deformed or doesn't move normally. Strains, sprains, and even some minor ankle fractures will heal well with home treatment.

During sports the knee is more likely to experience twisting and side contact—and injury. Abnormal motion is an important sign of knee injuries. Compare the injured knee to its opposite to get an idea of normal motion. Here are the signs of trouble:

- When ligaments tear, pain is intense immediately and subsides over time. Swelling is often quick and obvious. You may be able to wiggle the lower leg from side to side, or slide the knee from front to back. Torn knee ligaments usually need surgical repair as soon as possible.

- With torn knee cartilage, you may not be able to straighten the knee. Torn cartilage doesn't require immediate surgery, but deserves medical attention.

- Fractures affecting the knee area are less common than ankle injuries. They always need a doctor's care.

HOME TREATMENT

You can remember the best care for limb injuries with the word RIP—rest, ice, and protection.

- **Rest** the injury and keep it elevated.
- **Ice** wrapped in a towel applied to the injury for at least 30 minutes will help relieve pain and reduce swelling. If the joint is still painful, for the next several hours apply ice for 30 minutes and then leave it off for 15 minutes.

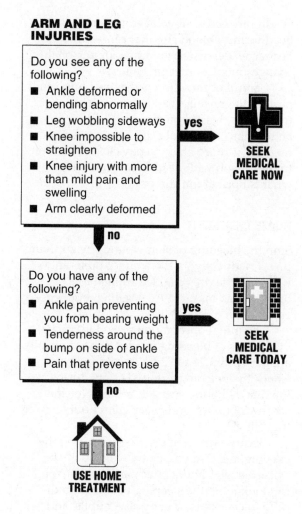

ARM AND LEG INJURIES

Do you see any of the following?
- Ankle deformed or bending abnormally
- Leg wobbling sideways
- Knee impossible to straighten
- Knee injury with more than mild pain and swelling
- Arm clearly deformed

yes → **SEEK MEDICAL CARE NOW**

no ↓

Do you have any of the following?
- Ankle pain preventing you from bearing weight
- Tenderness around the bump on side of ankle
- Pain that prevents use

yes → **SEEK MEDICAL CARE TODAY**

no ↓

USE HOME TREATMENT

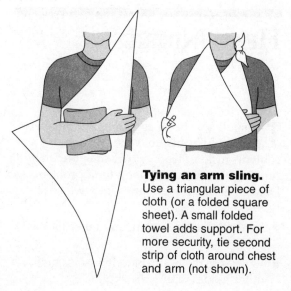

Tying an arm sling. Use a triangular piece of cloth (or a folded square sheet). A small folded towel adds support. For more security, tie second strip of cloth around chest and arm (not shown).

- **Protect** yourself by not putting weight on the injured joint. Obey the signals of pain; if something hurts, don't do it.

You can apply heat 24 hours after the injury. After 72 hours, the joint should begin to look, feel, and move normally again. If an injured knee remains painful and swollen despite rest, see the doctor.

An elastic bandage wrapped around the injured area can provide support but does not prevent reinjury (p. 155). Don't stretch the bandage tightly; this can cut off circulation. Don't use elastic bandages on children.

A sprain or strain can take four to six weeks to heal. Protect yourself by avoiding activities that may reinjure the joint.

WHAT TO EXPECT

The doctor will examine the joint for abnormal motion and ask about the quality of pain. He or she may order X-rays.

Using a needle, the doctor may remove blood from a massively swollen knee. A completely torn ligament may require surgery. In case of a fracture, a cast may be necessary to hold the bones in place while they heal. A sling can support an injured arm, if needed.

For injuries that appear minor, the doctor may advise you to continue home treatment. The doctor may give you pain medication, but acetaminophen is usually enough.

HEAD INJURIES

The skull is a strong container that protects and carefully cushions the valuable contents inside. Head injuries are potentially serious, but few lead to long-term problems. Doctors divide head injuries into two basic types:

- Injury to the bone, skin, and other tissues of the skull
- Injuries to the brain, blood vessels, and other tissues within the skull

Treat cuts, abrasions, and other wounds of the head as you would other trauma to the skin (p. 12). See the doctor if you suspect fracture of a skull bone, or if you see blood or clear fluid in the ears or nose following head injury.

A head injury that causes concussion or loss of consciousness requires **emergency** care. See the doctor as well if there may be bleeding or severe bruising within the head, suggested by these signs:

- Loss of alertness: increasing lethargy, unresponsiveness, abnormally deep sleep, coma
- Unequal pupil size after head injury (though about one in four people has slightly unequal pupils all the time)
- Severe vomiting or "projectile vomiting," which may be ejected several feet

In severe head injury, two or more signs are often present at once. Vomiting is usually forceful, repeated, and progressively worse.

In rare cases, slow bleeding inside the head forms a blood clot that causes chronic headache, persistent vomiting, or personality changes months after the injury.

Careful observation is the most important part of diagnosing head injury. You can usually do this at home as well as, if not better than, a hospital staff member. A family member is more likely to pay closer attention to the person with head injury and know what is normal for him or her.

HOME TREATMENT

Stop the bleeding of skin wounds by applying pressure directly on the wound, preferably with a sterile dressing. Ice applied to a bruised area may reduce swelling, but "goose eggs" often form anyway.

The initial observation period is crucial. Symptoms of bleeding inside the head usually appear within 24 to 72 hours after injury. Check the person every two hours during the first 24 hours, every four hours for the second 24 hours, and every eight hours for the third day.

Because many injuries occur during the evening, the injured person will usually be asleep several hours after the accident. You can look in on the sleeping person periodically to check his or her pulse, pupils, and arousability. If the person has a minor head bump and no sign of brain injury, nighttime checking is usually not necessary.

WHAT TO EXPECT

The doctor will ask about the nature of the accident and assess the patient's appearance and vital signs. He or she will do a physical exam and check for other injuries. If internal bleeding is possible, the patient may be kept

HEAD INJURIES

Have you seen any of the following signs?

- Unconsciousness
- Victim cannot remember injury
- Seizure
- Visual problems
- Bleeding from eyes, ears, or mouth
- Changes in behavior (irritability, lethargy, sleep)
- Fluid draining from nose
- Persistent vomiting
- Irregular breathing or heartbeat
- Child under two years of age, or possibly being abused
- Victim under influence of alcohol or drugs

yes → **SEEK MEDICAL CARE NOW**

no ↓

Is there a cut?

yes → *See:* Cuts and Scrapes (p. 12)

no ↓

USE HOME TREATMENT

in the hospital for observation. The doctor will avoid giving drugs, such as sedatives or strong pain medication, that may hide signs.

Bleeding within the skull is hard to diagnose. Skull X-rays are seldom helpful. CT scans and MRIs can be helpful but are expensive and may miss early accumulations of blood. With severe injuries, the victim may require X-rays of the neck to check for possible injury to the cervical spine.

BROKEN BONES?

You may find it hard to tell a broken bone from an injury to soft tissues, such as ligaments and tendons. Like a sprain or a strain, fractures are very painful. In most cases, the bone fragments remain aligned after the fracture, so you can't tell by sight whether a bone is broken; usually, neither can a doctor.

Besides obvious deformity of a limb (which requires medical attention), here are some signs of a serious fracture:

- If the fracture injures nearby nerves or blood vessels, a limb can be cold, pale, or numb—signs to call the doctor.
- Paleness, sweating, dizziness, and thirst are signs of shock. The person with these **emergency** signs needs immediate medical attention (p. 4).
- Sprains and other soft-tissue injuries usually allow some use of a limb, but fractures are often more disabling. While sprains and strains improve over a day or two, a broken bone may remain painful and unable to bear weight.
- Although soft-tissue injuries cause bruises under the skin, major bruising is more likely with a fracture.

Fortunately, few fractures are emergencies. In most fractures the bone pieces are in place and don't require setting. No harm is done if you wait a day or two before the doctor puts a cast on a broken arm or leg. After all, the cast doesn't cause healing; it just keeps the bones in place as they heal.

For broken ribs you can't do much more than tape and rest the affected ribs. If you have shortness of breath after chest injury, you may have hurt a lung. See the doctor right away.

For possible skull fracture, see Head Injuries (p. 20).

HOME TREATMENT

An ice pack on the injured area will help reduce pain and swelling. Rest and protect the limb for at least 48 hours.

Splinting an injured limb is a good way to rest the bone, especially if you are taking the person for medical care. Here are some guidelines for splinting:

- Immobilize the joints above and below the painful area. For example, to splint an injury of the lower arm, you must stop the elbow and wrist from moving.
- You can use any stiff material as a splint—a piece of wood, folded magazine, umbrella, or a rolled-up newspaper.
- Don't wrap the limb so tightly that you cut off circulation.

After 48 hours of rest, carefully test the limb. See if you can use it and whether it is

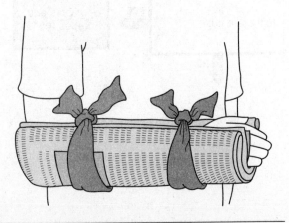

BROKEN BONE?

Do you see any of these signs?

- Limb is cold, blue, or numb
- Pelvis or thigh might be broken
- Victim is sweaty, pale, dizzy, or thirsty
- Limb is crooked

yes →

SEEK MEDICAL CARE NOW

↓ **no**

Do you see any of these signs?

- Limb that can't bear weight or be used
- A lot of bleeding and bruising in the injured area
- Fracture near a joint in a child

yes →

SEEK MEDICAL CARE TODAY

↓ **no**

USE HOME TREATMENT

Splints. Splinting keeps a limb from shifting as you apply home treatment or go to the hospital. *Left:* Forearm splint made of rolled newspaper and cloths. *Right:* A board wrapped in a towel used as a leg splint.

painful when moved. See the doctor for any injury that is still painful.

Take acetaminophen, aspirin, ibuprofen, or naproxen for pain.

WHAT TO EXPECT

A technician or assistant usually takes an X-ray of the injured area before you see the doctor. A crooked limb must be set, or straightened, which may require general anesthesia. The doctor may put pins in the bone during surgery to hold pieces together as they heal.

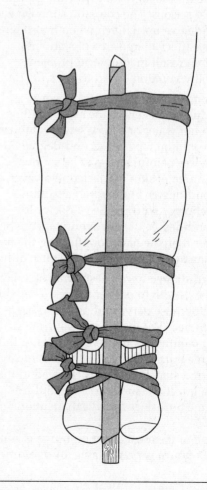

BURNS

Burns are injuries caused most commonly by heat. They can also result from chemicals, electricity, or radiation.

Heat burns are ranked according to the depth of skin injury:

- **First-degree burns** are superficial, resulting in red and tender skin. They are painful but rarely serious. The common sunburn is a first-degree burn. Even when first-degree burns affect a large area of skin, they seldom result in long-term problems. Usually you don't need to see a doctor.

- **Second-degree burns** are deeper, producing blisters of the skin. Scalding with hot water or a very severe sunburn are common types of second-degree burns. They are painful and may be serious if a large area of skin is affected. However, second-degree burns rarely result in infection or scarring. See a doctor for second-degree burns covering an area larger than the hand, or affecting the face or hands. Otherwise treat the burn at home.

- **Third-degree burns** destroy all skin layers and extend into deeper tissues. They do not hurt because nerve endings have been destroyed (but they may be surrounded by a painful second-degree burn). A third-degree burn usually involves obviously charred skin. Such burns can lead to fluid loss, infection, and scarring. All third-degree burns need medical attention.

One of the most common burns is sunburn. Sunburn is preventable, by avoiding tanning salons or prolonged exposure to the sun, and by using a sunscreen (p. 156).

Sunburn is most painful six to 48 hours after sun exposure. Injured skin may peel three to ten days after the burn. In rare cases, people with sunburn have visual problems. If this happens, call your doctor. Otherwise you don't need to see the doctor for a sunburn unless there is very severe pain or blistering.

HOME TREATMENT

For heat burns, immediately apply cold water or ice to the affected area. This stops the burning, limits the injury, and eases pain. Cool running water is fine. Apply cold until pain is relieved, or for about an hour. But do not apply cold so long that the burned area becomes numb. Reapply cold if needed.

For sunburn, cool compresses or cool oatmeal baths (Aveeno, etc.) may be helpful. Ordinary baking soda (one-half cup in a tub of water) is just as useful.

Anesthetic creams and sprays can relieve pain, but they may also slow healing, and they can cause irritation or allergic reactions in some people. Antibiotic creams such as Neosporin or Bacitracin probably do no harm to a burn, but they won't help a lot either. Don't apply butter, cream, or ointments such as Vaseline.

Use a pain reliever (p. 149).

Don't break blisters. If blisters break by themselves, leave the overlying skin in place. Keep the area clean, and protect yourself against the cause of blisters next time.

A burn that is painful for more than 48 hours requires medical attention.

WHAT TO EXPECT

The doctor will assess the size and severity of the burn and determine whether the victim

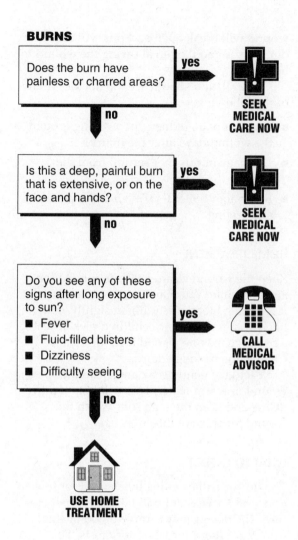

BURNS

Does the burn have painless or charred areas? — **yes** → **SEEK MEDICAL CARE NOW**

↓ **no**

Is this a deep, painful burn that is extensive, or on the face and hands? — **yes** → **SEEK MEDICAL CARE NOW**

↓ **no**

Do you see any of these signs after long exposure to sun?
- Fever
- Fluid-filled blisters
- Dizziness
- Difficulty seeing

— **yes** → **CALL MEDICAL ADVISOR**

↓ **no**

USE HOME TREATMENT

needs antibiotics, hospitalization, or skin grafts. Pain relievers may be prescribed.

The doctor may apply a dressing and/or an antibacterial ointment. Change the dressing regularly according to directions. Check the burn often for signs of infection.

Severe burns may require hospitalization. Third-degree burns may require skin grafts.

INFECTED WOUNDS

If a wound becomes infected, bacteria can grow in the bloodstream—a serious condition that doctors call "septicemia." This is why it's so important to clean a wound thoroughly and keep it clean.

Normally, after skin is hurt, the body begins to heal by forming a scab. These are the signs of *normal* healing:

- The wound may seep serum, which is yellowish and clear. (People often mistake serum for pus, which is thick, smelly, and never appears on the first day or so.)
- The edges of the wound will be pink or red.
- The wound may feel warm or itch.

The normal healing time depends on the type of wound. A minor wound requires about this amount of time:

- On the face—three to five days
- On the chest and arms—five to nine days
- On the legs—seven to twelve days

Larger wounds, or those that gape, requiring new skin or tissue to grow across an open space, need more time to heal. Children heal faster than adults. If a wound fails to heal within the expected time, call the doctor.

In contrast, an infected wound may fester within the skin, causing pain and swelling. Infection usually takes two to three days to develop. If you have an infection, it's a good idea for a doctor to examine the wound unless it is clearly minor. Sometimes a festering wound will break open and pus will drain out. This is good, often allowing the wound to heal well.

Overall, you should see the doctor for any of the following:

- A rise in pain, redness, or swelling around the wound days after the injury
- Drainage of pus (not serum) from the wound
- Fever above 99.9°F (37.7°C) and a general sick feeling

HOME TREATMENT

Keep the wound clean. Leave it open to the air if possible. You may bandage the wound if it is oozing blood or serum, unsightly, or likely to get dirty. Since children pick at scabs, a bandage may be a good idea for them. Change the bandage daily.

Each day gently soak and clean the wound in warm water. This will help remove debris and keep the scab soft. Watch the wound for signs of infection.

WHAT TO EXPECT

The doctor will examine the wound for infection, and an assistant will take your temperature. The doctor may sample blood or fluid from the wound for laboratory tests. The doctor may prescribe antibiotics.

If the wound is festering, the doctor may drain it with a needle or scalpel. This is not very painful and actually relieves discomfort.

For severe infections you may need to stay in the hospital.

INFECTED WOUNDS

Are any of the following present?
- Fever above 99.9°F (37.7°C) and a general ill feeling
- An increase of pain, redness, or swelling a day or more after the injury
- Thick, smelly pus draining from the wound

yes →

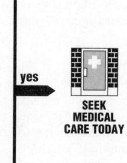

SEEK MEDICAL CARE TODAY

no ↓

USE HOME TREATMENT

TETANUS SHOTS

Tetanus (lockjaw) is caused by a germ that can grow inside a wound if dirt or foreign bodies become lodged beneath the skin. Puncture wounds are more likely to become infected than cuts caused by sharp, clean objects such as knives or razor blades. Abrasions and minor burns don't result in tetanus.

Usually people receive a series of tetanus shots and boosters during childhood. After a full series of five shots there is immunity for at least ten years. You should have a booster if a wound has left foreign debris beneath the skin and isn't open to the air, and if you haven't had a tetanus shot within the past ten years. Call your doctor if you never received the basic series of shots or are unsure of your immunization status.

Tetanus immunization is very important. The tetanus germ is quite common and the disease is severe. Be sure each of your children has the basic series of shots and boosters. Keep a record of your family's immunizations.

VIRUS, BACTERIA, OR ALLERGY?

When an upper respiratory illness strikes you, the first question is whether a virus, bacteria, or allergy is causing it. The doctor can cure a bacterial infection with an antibiotic. However, viral infections and allergies have no cure.

For the most part, allergies and viral illnesses get better on their own. Doctors manage them by relieving the *symptoms* while nature takes its course. An antibiotic could do more harm than good. In many cases you can manage the symptoms of viral illness and allergies as well as, if not better than, your doctor. A doctor may prescribe treatment for allergies if home treatment fails.

Viral Syndromes

Viral illnesses generally have three basic patterns. You may have symptoms of more than one syndrome.

- **Upper respiratory infection,** the common cold: fever, sore throat, runny nose, congestion, stuffiness, hoarseness, swollen glands
- **Influenza,** the flu: high fever, severe headache, muscle aches and pain
- **Gastroenteritis,** stomach flu: nausea, vomiting, diarrhea, and crampy abdominal pain

Hay Fever

Allergic rhinitis, or hay fever, is the most common allergy problem. Symptoms include stuffy, runny nose; watering, itchy eyes; headache; and sneezing. Common sources of allergies are pollens and dust. The best prevention is to avoid or reduce substances that trigger allergies.

Sinusitis

The sinuses often get inflamed when you have hay fever or asthma. Symptoms include a feeling of fullness, heaviness, or pressure behind the nose and eyes, often producing a sinus headache. You may also have a fever and nasal discharge. Antihistamines and decongestants (p. 146) may help. Don't use nasal sprays (p. 146) for more than three days in a row. See your doctor if sinusitis recurs.

Strep Throat

The streptococcus bacterium can cause a painful infection of the throat. Symptoms include sore throat, fever, swollen lymph glands in the neck, and sometimes abdominal pain. The person with strep throat may also have a red rash on the face and along the creases of the elbow, armpit, and knee—signs of scarlet fever. Doctors treat strep throat with antibiotics. You should have it diagnosed and treated early.

Other Conditions

Many other factors play a role in upper respiratory disorders. Smoking is the largest single cause of coughs and sore throats. Air pollution is another common problem. Tumors and other serious diseases are rare by comparison. Talk to your doctor about symptoms that last for more than two weeks.

Virus, Bacteria, or Allergy?

	Virus	Bacteria	Allergy
Runny nose?	Often	Rare	Often
Aching muscles?	Usual	Rare	Never
Headache (non-sinus)?	Often	Rare	Never
Dizzy?	Often	Rare	Rare
Fever?	Often	Often	Never
Cough?	Often	Sometimes	Rare
Dry cough?	Often	Rare	Sometimes
Raising sputum?	Rare	Often	Rare
Hoarseness?	Often	Rare	Sometimes
Recurs at a particular season?	No	No	Often
Do antibiotics help?	No	Yes	No
Can the doctor help?	Seldom	Yes	Sometimes

COLDS AND FLU

The common cold and the different kinds of flu account for more unnecessary visits to the doctor than any other illness.

Because viruses cause colds and the flu, the doctor can't cure them with an antibiotic or any other drug. Usually you can care for your symptoms as well as the doctor. Nonprescription drugs—pain relievers, decongestants, and antihistamines—can relieve your symptoms while your body recovers.

Read the appropriate section of this book for information about specific symptoms, such as Ear Problems (p. 34), Sore Throat (p. 32), Cough (p. 36), Nausea and Vomiting (p. 88), and Diarrhea (p. 90). The doctor can help if you develop an ear infection (p. 34) or bacterial pneumonia. A very young child with a viral infection needs medical attention.

A runny nose is an important sign that the body is trying to rid itself of cold or flu viruses. Sneezes are another way the nose removes germs and other irritants. Unfortunately, sneezes are also one way that viruses pass from person to person. Cover your nose and mouth with a tissue or handkerchief when you sneeze. Wash your hands often when you have a runny nose or sneeze; cold and flu viruses are spread most often by direct contact.

Complications from a runny nose are due to the excess mucus. The mucus can run into the throat (postnasal drip) and cause a sore throat or a cough that is most obvious at night. Mucus drip can block the eustachian tube between the nasal passages and the ear, resulting in ear infection and pain. It can also lead to infection and pain in the sinuses.

A runny nose can also be a sign of other conditions:

- **Allergies** Hay fever (allergic rhinitis) can cause the nose to run clear, very thin mucus. People with hay fever will often have other symptoms, including sneezing and itching, and watery eyes. Hay fever lasts longer than a viral infection, often for weeks or months. Allergies are more common in the spring and fall, when pollen and other allergens are in the air. Other substances that can cause allergic rhinitis include house dust, mold, and animal dander.

- **Nose Sprays** Prolonged use of nose sprays or drops can lead to a runny nose. Nose drops containing substances like ephedrine should never be used for more than three consecutive days. You can avoid this problem by switching to saline nose drops for a few days.

- **Head Injury** Head injury is a rare but serious cause of a runny nose (p. 20). If a person has clear discharge that began after a head injury, he or she needs immediate medical attention.

HOME TREATMENT

You can take acetaminophen, aspirin, ibuprofen, or naproxen remedies (p. 149) for the fever and aches of the common cold. These symptoms are usually worse in the afternoon and evening, so take medications regularly during this time. Don't give aspirin to children or teenagers; give them acetaminophen instead.

There are two basic kinds of cold symptom remedies:

- Decongestants that shrink the nasal membranes and open the passages

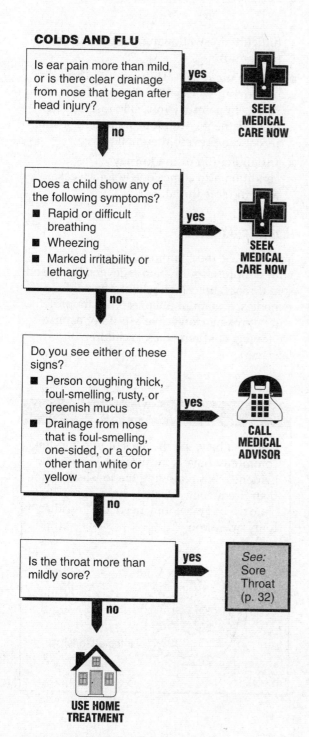

COLDS AND FLU

Is ear pain more than mild, or is there clear drainage from nose that began after head injury? — **yes** → **SEEK MEDICAL CARE NOW**

no ↓

Does a child show any of the following symptoms?
- Rapid or difficult breathing
- Wheezing
- Marked irritability or lethargy

yes → **SEEK MEDICAL CARE NOW**

no ↓

Do you see either of these signs?
- Person coughing thick, foul-smelling, rusty, or greenish mucus
- Drainage from nose that is foul-smelling, one-sided, or a color other than white or yellow

yes → **CALL MEDICAL ADVISOR**

no ↓

Is the throat more than mildly sore? — **yes** → *See:* Sore Throat (p. 32)

no ↓

USE HOME TREATMENT

- Antihistamines that reduce secretions in the nose

Save money and have fewer side effects by matching the remedy to your symptoms.

Drink a lot of liquid. The body requires more fluid when you have a fever. Fluids help to keep the mucus more liquid and to prevent complications such as bronchitis and ear infection. A vaporizer, particularly in the winter, can help as well.

Blowing your nose makes you feel better and offers the advantage of safely moving mucus, virus particles, and allergens outside the body. Sniffing a runny nose increases your risk of ear infection.

Call the doctor if symptoms last more than two weeks.

WHAT TO EXPECT

The doctor will take the history and do a physical examination. He or she may order a chest X-ray or swab the nose or throat for laboratory analysis.

The doctor may prescribe a decongestant or antihistamine. If you have a bacterial infection, the doctor may prescribe an antibiotic. If you suffer from allergies, the doctor may advise you how to reduce your exposure to pollen and other triggers.

SORE THROAT

Sore throat can affect a person of any age but is most common among children five to ten years old. One cause is breathing through the mouth, which can dry and irritate the air passages; this irritation improves quickly when moist air is breathed. The most common causes of sore throat, however, are viruses and bacteria.

Antibiotics are useless against viral infection. A sore throat caused by virus must improve on its own. Pain relievers, throat lozenges, anesthetic sprays, and other medications may relieve symptoms.

Infectious mononucleosis, also called "mono" or "the kissing disease," is a viral sore throat common among older children and adolescents. The person with mono may have a severe sore throat for more than a week, and feel particularly weak.

"Strep throat" is what we commonly call sore throat caused by a streptococcal bacterium. Strep throat is more common in children than adults. If one child in a family has strep throat, other members with a sore throat are likely also to be infected with strep.

A sore throat is unlikely to be strep if the person has several other cold symptoms: runny nose, stuffy ears, cough, and so on.

You should have a strep throat diagnosed and treated with antibiotics as soon as possible to avoid rare but serious complications, such as:

- **Throat abscess** Suspect a throat abscess if a child drools excessively or has great difficulty in swallowing or opening his or her mouth.

- **Rheumatic fever** This condition appears one to four weeks after the sore throat and results in painful joints, skin rashes, and heart damage. Antibiotic treatment of strep throat can prevent rheumatic fever.

- **Inflammation of the kidney** This condition also comes one to four weeks after the sore throat.

HOME TREATMENT

You can ease the symptoms of sore throat with nonprescription pain relievers. Fever and sore throat pain can be relieved by cold remedies, acetaminophen, aspirin, ibuprofen, and naproxen. Don't give aspirin or aspirin-containing cold remedies to children or teenagers.

TONSIL PROBLEMS

Children between the ages of five and ten commonly have sore throats. There is no evidence that removing the tonsils lowers their frequency. Doctors now agree that children very seldom need the tonsillectomy operation.

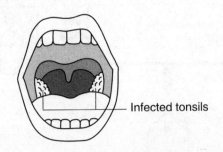

Infected tonsils

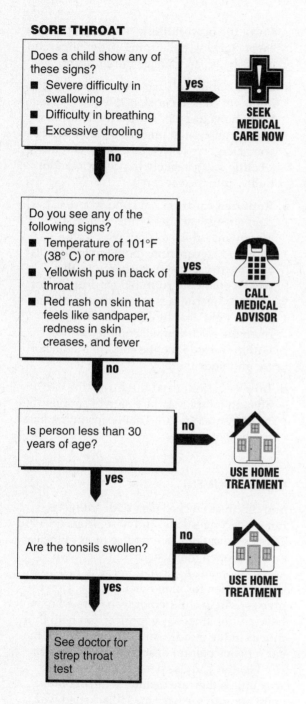

SORE THROAT

Does a child show any of these signs?
- Severe difficulty in swallowing
- Difficulty in breathing
- Excessive drooling

yes → SEEK MEDICAL CARE NOW

no ↓

Do you see any of the following signs?
- Temperature of 101°F (38° C) or more
- Yellowish pus in back of throat
- Red rash on skin that feels like sandpaper, redness in skin creases, and fever

yes → CALL MEDICAL ADVISOR

no ↓

Is person less than 30 years of age?

no → USE HOME TREATMENT

yes ↓

Are the tonsils swollen?

no → USE HOME TREATMENT

yes ↓

See doctor for strep throat test

A vaporizer will moisten the air and ease dry air passages. Saltwater gargles or tea with honey or lemon also may help. Your symptoms will improve over time.

WHAT TO EXPECT

The doctor may do a "quick test" for strep, or swab the throat for lab tests. Some doctors delay prescribing an antibiotic until they know the results of culture tests. A delay of treatment by a day or two doesn't increase the risk of rheumatic fever.

The doctor may prescribe antibiotics, which treat a bacterial infection and prevent complications but don't ease throat discomfort. Antibiotics are useless against sore throat caused by virus.

EAR PROBLEMS

When you have a cold or allergy, the eustachian tube between the middle ear and the nasal passages can swell and close off. Fluid, unable to drain through the eustachian tube, then backs up behind the eardrum. The buildup of pressure causes stuffiness, decreased hearing, and pain. This is most common in small children. The fluid behind the eardrum is also a good medium for bacteria.

You may also feel ear pain and stuffiness at higher altitudes, such as during air travel. Here are some ways to keep the eustachian tubes open in such situations:

- Swallow and chew gum as the pressure changes.
- Young children can drink from a bottle or use a pacifier.
- Close your mouth and pinch your nostrils shut while pretending to blow your nose.
- Use a decongestant before traveling if you anticipate problems.

Fever and pain, often in one ear, are signs of ear infection. Children may show other symptoms, such as fussiness, increased crying, irritability, and pulling at the ears. Children rarely have permanent hearing loss from an ear infection.

Less common ear problems include:

- **Swimmer's ear**   This inflammation of the outer ear and canal is common in the summer. Its symptoms include ear discharge, redness, itchiness, and pain.

Resist the powerful urge to scratch the ear canal. Sticking in hairpins, paper clips, and other items can damage the eardrum.

- **Ear wax buildup**   Ear wax, a protective lining for the ear canal, is rarely a problem. Washing your outer ear during bathing is usually enough to prevent the buildup of wax. Don't try to clean the inner ear; using a cotton swab is likely to pack wax more tightly into the ear canal.

- **Ruptured eardrum**   A child whose ear pain goes away after white, yellow, or bloody material leaks out may have ruptured an eardrum. (Sometimes parents find the dry, crusted discharge on the child's pillow.) A ruptured eardrum is not cause for alarm. It is a natural part of the body's fight against ear infection. Most often the eardrum will completely heal within weeks. Take the child to the doctor for antibiotic therapy.

- **Injury**   Clear or red fluid from the ear after an injury may be a sign of serious head trauma (p. 20). That needs immediate medical attention.

HOME TREATMENT

You can treat blocked ears with antihistamines, decongestants, and nose drops (p. 146). These medications will reduce fluid in the ear and help open the eustachian tube. Give acetaminophen, aspirin, ibuprofen, naproxen, or ketoprofen for pain relief (p. 149). Don't give aspirin to children or teenagers who may have a viral illness. A vaporizer can help thin mucus in the middle ear. See the doctor if the ear remains painful despite home treatment.

We don't advise parents to remove ear wax unless they are dealing with an older child and can see hardened, blackened wax.

EAR PROBLEMS

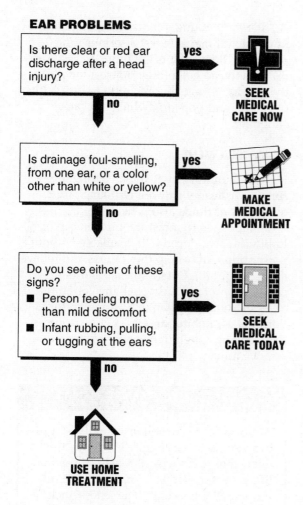

Is there clear or red ear discharge after a head injury?

yes → **SEEK MEDICAL CARE NOW**

no ↓

Is drainage foul-smelling, from one ear, or a color other than white or yellow?

yes → **MAKE MEDICAL APPOINTMENT**

no ↓

Do you see either of these signs?
- Person feeling more than mild discomfort
- Infant rubbing, pulling, or tugging at the ears

yes → **SEEK MEDICAL CARE TODAY**

no ↓

USE HOME TREATMENT

Here are tips for softening the wax and flushing the ear with liquid:

- Never flush the ear with water if the eardrum may be hurt or damaged.
- You can soften ear wax with olive oil. Over-the-counter remedies, such as Debrox and Cerumenex, may irritate the ear; read the directions carefully.

- When flushing the ear, use water as close to body temperature as possible.
- Flush the ear gently with a bulb syringe, available at the drug store, or a water jet (e.g., Water Pik) at the *lowest* setting; higher settings may damage the ear.

You can often treat swimmer's ear at home. Soak a piece of cotton with Burow's solution and place it in the ear canal overnight. If you can't find Burow's solution at your pharmacy, mix enough Merthiolate in mineral oil to turn it pink, and use this to soak the cotton. In the morning, use a bulb syringe to flush the ear with 3% hydrogen peroxide solution, followed by tepid water. See the doctor if symptoms last more than two weeks.

WHAT TO EXPECT

The doctor will take the history and do a physical examination, looking particularly at the ears, nose, and throat. If you have any discharge from the ear, the doctor may take a sample for laboratory analysis.

If you have signs of an ear infection, the doctor may prescribe antibiotics, antihistamines, and drops (p. 146). If you have an ear canal inflammation, the doctor may prescribe ear drops or a therapy described in the home treatment section. Take all medication as directed.

Occasionally, fluid persists in the middle ear even when there isn't an infection. This can lead to hearing loss. If the condition persists, the doctor may suggest the insertion of a tube into the eardrum to drain the middle ear. This is a simple, effective, and common procedure.

COUGH

The cough reflex is one of the body's best defenses. The violent rush of air clears foreign material from the air passages. Smoke, air pollutants, accidentally inhaled food, or any other airway irritation can trigger a cough.

When you have a cold, mucus from the nasal passages may drain into the airway (postnasal drip) and trigger the cough reflex. You can treat this with a cough suppressant.

If your lungs are congested, coughing may expel pus and mucus. This type of "productive" cough is helpful in clearing the lungs. You should not suppress a productive cough with drugs.

Here are some of the common causes of cough:

- **Smoking** kills the cells lining the airway so that you can't expel mucus normally. The smoker's chronic cough is evidence of the continual irritation of the air passages.

- **Viral infections** can cause a cough that usually produces yellow or white mucus. Antibiotics are useless to treat a viral infection. The illness runs its course within a few days.

- **Bacterial infections** can cause a cough that usually produces rusty or green mucus. The mucus looks like it contains pus. Your doctor can prescribe an antibiotic to treat a bacterial infection. Doctors use the term "pneumonia" most often to mean a bacterial infection of the lung, but the same label can be applied to other lung infections, more or less serious. Don't panic if you hear that word.

For very young infants, coughing is unusual and may suggest a serious lung problem. Older infants are prone to swallow things and can get a foreign object lodged in the airway. Young children tend to inhale bits of peanut and popcorn, which can cause coughing.

HOME TREATMENT

Increase humidity by using a vaporizer or running a steamy shower. Drinking large quantities of fluids also is helpful.

In addition to moisture, guaifenesin (e.g., Robitussin, Naldecon CX), available without a prescription, may help thin mucus and relieve a cough (p. 147). Cough lozenges or hard candy may relieve a dry, tickling cough.

Dextromethorphan (e.g., Romilar, Vicks Formula 44, Robitussin-DM) helps suppress a dry, hacking cough that is not helping to remove mucus (p. 147).

HOARSENESS

A vocal cord problem usually causes hoarseness or laryngitis. In adults, this is often due to a virus; the hoarseness may linger after other symptoms resolve. Causes of persistent hoarseness include cigarette smoke, overusing your voice, cysts on the vocal cords, or even cancer. If you are a smoker, stop smoking and wait one month. See the doctor if you're still hoarse.

Hoarseness in young infants may be due to a birth defect or other medical condition. In young children, hoarseness is usually due to excessive crying, which strains the vocal cords. Viral infection is the most common cause of hoarseness in older children.

COUGH AND HOARSENESS

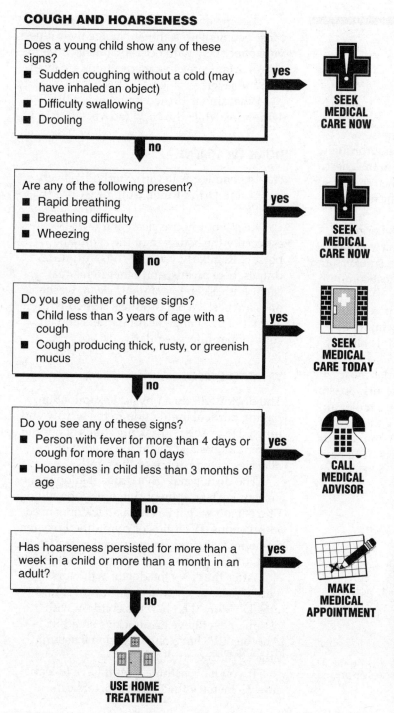

Does a young child show any of these signs?
- Sudden coughing without a cold (may have inhaled an object)
- Difficulty swallowing
- Drooling

yes → **SEEK MEDICAL CARE NOW**

no ↓

Are any of the following present?
- Rapid breathing
- Breathing difficulty
- Wheezing

yes → **SEEK MEDICAL CARE NOW**

no ↓

Do you see either of these signs?
- Child less than 3 years of age with a cough
- Cough producing thick, rusty, or greenish mucus

yes → **SEEK MEDICAL CARE TODAY**

no ↓

Do you see any of these signs?
- Person with fever for more than 4 days or cough for more than 10 days
- Hoarseness in child less than 3 months of age

yes → **CALL MEDICAL ADVISOR**

no ↓

Has hoarseness persisted for more than a week in a child or more than a month in an adult?

yes → **MAKE MEDICAL APPOINTMENT**

no ↓

USE HOME TREATMENT

Decongestants and/or antihistamines can help if postnasal drip is causing the cough. Otherwise avoid antihistamines because they dry and thicken secretions.

Unless a cold or other illness causes it, hoarseness may be difficult to treat. Rest the vocal cords; crying or shouting makes them worse. Humidifying the air can help. Healing may take several days as nature takes its course.

WHAT TO EXPECT

The doctor will take the history and do a physical exam. He or she may order a chest X-ray or blood tests. In some cases of hoarseness, the doctor may look at the vocal cords with the help of a small mirror.

If you have a cough that over-the-counter remedies have not helped, the doctor may prescribe medication. Doctors don't usually prescribe antibiotics for a cough or hoarseness.

HICCUPS

For hiccups, research suggests that the most effective treatment is one-half teaspoon (3 ml) of dry sugar placed on the back of the tongue.

WHEEZING

Wheezing is a high-pitched noise or whistle caused by air flowing through narrowed breathing tubes deep in the chest. Wheezing is usually obvious when the person breathes out, but you may also hear it when he or she breathes in.

Viral infection, pneumonia, allergic reaction, or foreign matter in the airway can cause wheezing. It is common in smokers and people with emphysema. The most common reason for wheezing is asthma.

All wheezing in children is potentially serious. A wheezing child needs immediate medical attention unless a doctor is already treating him or her for asthma.

Asthma is a breathing disorder most common in children and adolescents. Spasm and excessive mucus narrow the smaller air passages in the lung, obstructing the flow of air and resulting in wheezing. Asthma tends to run in families where members have hay fever or eczema. An attack may be triggered by:

- Viral or bacterial infection
- Emotional stress
- Cold air
- Air pollution
- Allergic reaction to house dust, pollen, mold, food, animal dander, and other things
- New medication

Most often, there's no clear reason for an asthmatic attack.

Asthma and viral illnesses have no cure. Most people with asthma manage their illness very effectively with occasional help from the doctor. Many effective medications are available for severe problems.

Wheezing is treated by relieving the symptoms while the body recovers.

HOME TREATMENT

Having enough water in your body is very important. Drink water, fruit juices, or soft drinks.

Keep your house clean and dust-free, especially the bedroom of the asthmatic person. Regularly vacuum rugs, furniture, drapes, bedspreads, and other items that catch dust. Keep toy animals clean; washable ones are best. Avoid products stuffed with animal hair. Change heating filters and air conditioner filters regularly.

WHAT TO EXPECT

The doctor will do a physical examination, paying particular attention to the airway and lungs. He or she will ask questions about the current illness and about the history of allergies in the patient or the family.

The doctor may give drugs that open the airway, such as epinephrine or theophylline. The person with an asthma attack may need intravenous (IV) fluids or humidified oxygen. Sometimes the person may need to stay in the hospital for observation and treatment.

After the crisis the doctor will work with you to manage asthma and prevent future attacks. More than half the children with asthma never have an attack as an adult. Another 10% have only occasional asthma attacks during adult life.

If you have asthma, you'll have to learn how to manage the illness. Doctors can

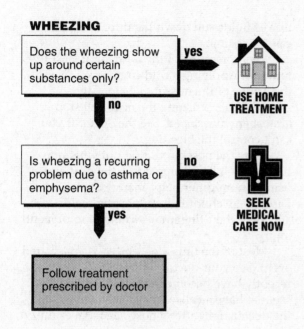

WHEEZING

Does the wheezing show up around certain substances only? **yes** → **USE HOME TREATMENT**

no ↓

Is wheezing a recurring problem due to asthma or emphysema? **no** → **SEEK MEDICAL CARE NOW**

yes ↓

Follow treatment prescribed by doctor

prescribe several medications to help you; avoid drugs that combine ingredients because of added side effects. Avoid antihistamines, which can dry out your airway. Talk to your doctor before using corticosteroid drugs such as prednisone. Learn how to use such devices as a nebulizer or a metered-dose inhaler properly.

NOSEBLEEDS

The nose has thin membranes that are rich with blood vessels. They can start to bleed after a minor injury, vigorous nose-blowing, or even an irritating cold virus.

Nosebleeds are more common during the winter, when indoor air is dry and heated. In children, picking the nose is a common cause of bleeding.

Some doctors believe high blood pressure can cause nosebleeds. If you have high blood pressure and have a nosebleed, talk to your doctor about having your blood pressure measured soon.

Remember these key points:

- You can almost always stop nosebleeds yourself.
- Colds or minor nose injury causes most nosebleeds.
- Packing the nose with gauze has significant drawbacks.
- Even when recurring nosebleeds mean you should see a doctor, the appointment is not urgent; it's easier to diagnose the problem after the bleeding stops.

HOME TREATMENT

The nose has a soft part and a bony, hard part. Nosebleeds usually happen in the soft part. Squeezing the soft portion of the nose between the thumb and forefinger can control these nosebleeds.

Have the person with nosebleed sit and pinch the nose. Don't tip the head back—this makes fluids run down the throat and can cause gagging.

Keep pressure on the nose for at least five minutes. Applying a cold compress or ice to the bridge of the nose may help. Given enough time, pinching the nose will stop almost any nosebleed. See the doctor if you can't control the bleeding.

After the nosebleed, find out what may have caused it. Turning down the heat and using a humidifier helps many people. Discourage children from picking their noses, and keep their fingernails trimmed to prevent injury.

Most of the time a nosebleed is an isolated event. See your doctor if nosebleeds recur, recently have become more frequent, or don't seem to have a cause. You don't need to see the doctor right after a nosebleed. An examination may start the nose bleeding again.

WHAT TO EXPECT

If home treatment fails to control a nosebleed, the doctor will examine the nose to find the source of bleeding. He or she may seal the bleeding area with electrical or chemical cauterization. If that doesn't work, the doctor may put packing in the nasal passage. In this case, the patient must be carefully observed to avoid infection.

If you're having recurring nosebleeds, the doctor may ask about events preceding the nosebleeds and do a thorough examination of the nose. Rarely, he or she may run tests to check blood clotting.

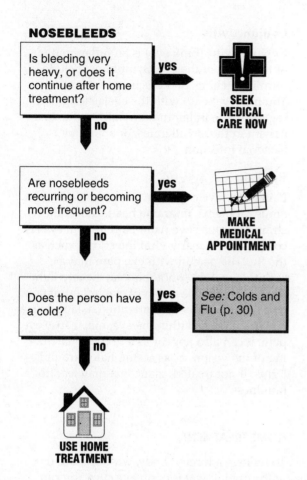

NOSEBLEEDS

Is bleeding very heavy, or does it continue after home treatment? — **yes** → **SEEK MEDICAL CARE NOW**

no ↓

Are nosebleeds recurring or becoming more frequent? — **yes** → **MAKE MEDICAL APPOINTMENT**

no ↓

Does the person have a cold? — **yes** → *See:* Colds and Flu (p. 30)

no ↓

USE HOME TREATMENT

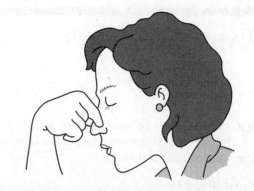

To stop a nosebleed. Sit down and squeeze just below the hard portion of the nose. Hold for five minutes. It isn't necessary to tilt the head back.

EYE CONDITIONS

You must take eye conditions seriously. See the doctor if you have any doubts or questions about your status.

Burst Blood Vessel

If a blood vessel in the white of the eye breaks, it may create an ugly red spot. This blood spot will go away in a few weeks. You can wait it out without seeing the doctor as long as only the white of the eye is affected and you have no vision problems or pain. Call the doctor if you're taking blood-thinning medications.

Foreign Body

A foreign body in the eye must be removed before it can cause vision problems. Seek medical attention if:

- The foreign body was thrown into the eye with force
- The foreign body was produced by metal striking metal; a small metal particle can penetrate the eyeball
- You can see blood in the eye

A minor foreign body, such as a grain of sand blown in by the wind, can usually be flushed out with tears.

Even after the foreign body is removed it can feel as if it is still in the eye. You may have scraped the cornea, the clear covering over the front of the eye. Cornea injuries usually heal quickly without problems.

See the doctor if you're still having symptoms after 48 hours.

Conjunctivitis

Conjunctivitis (pink eye) is an inflammation of the lining of the eye. Symptoms include burning, itching, and discharge from the eye. You may wake up with the eyelashes glued together. The inflammation may be due to an irritant in the air, allergies, or a viral or bacterial infection.

Eye Pain

Pain in the eye can be an important symptom. Sinus problems, migraine headache, and eye strain can cause eye pain. Pain in both eyes is common with many viral infections, such as the flu. The person with eye pain may be sensitive to light (photophobia). Severe light sensitivity may be a sign of eye inflammation that requires a doctor's attention. Glaucoma, a rise in pressure within the eye, may cause eye pain; it can also appear as a gradual narrowing of the vision, or as seeing halos around lights. If not treated, glaucoma may lead to blindness.

HOME TREATMENT

To remove a foreign body, wash the eye out with running water or an eye cup. You can use water, but a weak boric acid solution is better; read the directions on the package. Inspect the eye. Use a good light and shine it on the eye from both the front and the side. Have someone else inspect the eye as well. Don't rub the eye—you might scratch the cornea. An eye patch for the first 24 hours will help relieve pain. Make a patch by taping several layers of gauze in place over the eye. Check the eye every day by reading different sizes of newspaper type from across the room.

Conjunctivitis usually clears up within a few days if it is not caused by bacteria. Otherwise, washing the eye with a boric acid

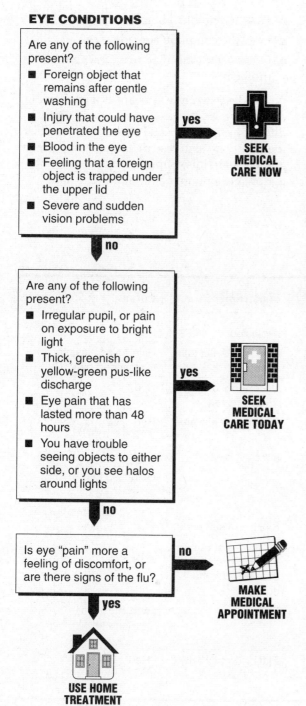

EYE CONDITIONS

Are any of the following present?

- Foreign object that remains after gentle washing
- Injury that could have penetrated the eye
- Blood in the eye
- Feeling that a foreign object is trapped under the upper lid
- Severe and sudden vision problems

yes → **SEEK MEDICAL CARE NOW**

no ↓

Are any of the following present?

- Irregular pupil, or pain on exposure to bright light
- Thick, greenish or yellow-green pus-like discharge
- Eye pain that has lasted more than 48 hours
- You have trouble seeing objects to either side, or you see halos around lights

yes → **SEEK MEDICAL CARE TODAY**

no ↓

Is eye "pain" more a feeling of discomfort, or are there signs of the flu?

no → **MAKE MEDICAL APPOINTMENT**

yes ↓

USE HOME TREATMENT

solution will help remove bacteria and debris; follow the directions carefully. Eye drops (e.g., Murine, Visine) may soothe bacterial conjunctivitis but won't cure it. See your doctor if the eye irritation doesn't clear up, if the discharge gets thicker, or if you have eye pain or a problem with vision.

For burning or itching eyes, identify the cause and eliminate it. Air conditioning in your home and car will help eliminate pollen and other irritants. You may find it useful to wear dark glasses and goggles at work. Avoid chlorinated swimming pools. Antihistamines may help if your problem is allergies.

You can take a pain reliever (p. 149) for mild eye discomfort from other causes. Dark glasses may help if your eyes are sensitive to light.

WHAT TO EXPECT

The doctor will check vision and examine the eyes. An ophthalmologist (eye surgeon) may do a slit-lamp examination; he or she may check the pressure within the eye, which is a quick and painless procedure.

If you have a foreign object in the eye, the doctor will drop a fluorescent dye into the eye and examine it under an ultraviolet light. You will have X-rays taken if the object may have penetrated the globe of the eye. The doctor will remove the foreign body with a cotton swab, eyewash solution, or a small needle. He or she may apply an antibiotic ointment and an eye patch.

The doctor may prescribe antihistamines for itchy, burning eyes. He or she may prescribe eye drops or ointment for conjunctivitis and other infections.

SKIN DISEASES

Doctors identify skin diseases by recognizing patterns in:

- How the skin looks now

- How the problem began
- How the condition spread
- Other symptoms that arrived with the skin problem

A skin disease rarely appears as a textbook case, however. Because every case is slightly different, even the best doctors won't be able to identify all skin diseases right away. The guidelines in this chapter allow for a reasonable amount of variation. The table

Skin Problems

	Fever	Itching	Elevation	Color
Diaper Rash	No	No	If infected	Red
Hives	No	Intense	Raised with flat tops	Pale, raised lesions surrounded by red
Eczema	No	Moderate to intense	Occasional blisters when infected	Red
Poison Ivy and Poison Oak	No	Intense	Blisters are elevated	Red
Acne	No	No	Pimples, cysts	Red
Athlete's Foot and Jock Itch (fungal infections)	No	Mild to intense	No	Colorless to red
Ringworm (fungal infection)	No	Occasionally	Slightly raised rings	Red
Chicken Pox (childhood illness)	Yes	Intense during crusty stage	Flat, then raised, then blisters, then crusts	Red
Measles (childhood illness)	Yes	None to mild	Flat	Pink, then red
Rubella (childhood illness)	Yes	No	Flat or slightly raised	Red

below will let you quickly review the major symptoms of common skin problems and point you in the right direction.

Often you'll have an idea what the problem is even before checking the table. Rashes are very common. After a while many people get pretty good at identifying ringworm, poison ivy, and other skin conditions. Don't be afraid to ask others for their opinions. Grandparents and others have seen a lot of skin problems over the years and know what they look like.

We've listed the most common skin problems, but by no means all. Call the doctor if your problem doesn't seem to fit these patterns and may be serious.

Fortunately, the vast majority of skin problems are minor, get better by themselves, and pose no risk to health. Usually you can wait a while to see if the problem goes away.

Skin Problems

	Location	Duration	Other Symptoms
Diaper Rash	Under diaper	Until controlled	
Hives	Anywhere	Minutes to days	
Eczema	Elbows, wrists, knees, cheeks	Until controlled	Moistness; oozing
Poison Ivy and Poison Oak	Exposed areas	7 to 14 days	Oozing; some swelling
Acne	Face, back, chest	Until controlled	Blackheads
Athlete's Foot and Jock Itch (fungal infections)	Between toes; in groin	Until controlled	Cracks; scaling; oozing blisters
Ringworm (fungal infection)	Anywhere, including scalp and nails	Until controlled	Flaking or scaling
Chicken Pox (childhood illness)	May start anywhere; most prominent on trunk and face	4 to 10 days	Lesions progress from flat to tiny blisters, then become crusted
Measles (childhood illness)	First face, then chest and abdomen, then arms and legs	4 to 7 days	Preceded by fever, cough, red eyes
Rubella (childhood illness)	First face, then trunk, then extremities	2 to 4 days	Swollen glands behind ears; joint pain in some older children and adults

HIVES

Hives, also called urticaria, are a rash that develops as an allergic reaction. The rash looks like small red bumps. The bumps may appear in clusters and are very itchy.

Just about anything can cause hives, including cold, heat, and even emotional tension. Among some more common causes of hives are:

- Drugs
- Eggs
- Milk and cheese
- Wheat
- Pork
- Seafood
- Berries
- Nuts
- Pollen
- Animal dander
- Insect bites

Allergy testing is the only way to tell for sure what is causing hives. A doctor will expose you to substances that may cause a reaction. If you react with hives, avoid the substances that seem to have caused the reaction.

A person who develops hives could at some point have a more severe systemic reaction, including breathing difficulty and shock. This is an **emergency.** Drive this person to the hospital immediately. If you're having the reaction yourself and have no other way to reach medical care, call for an ambulance rather than risk driving.

Fortunately, most people only have one attack of hives, lasting minutes to weeks. Often hives go away without therapy, as mysteriously as they came.

HOME TREATMENT

If you have hives, look for a pattern to their appearance. Do they appear after meals? After exposure to cold? During a particular time of the year? Eliminate possible causes and see what happens.

If hives developed after you took a dose of medication, call the doctor before taking another dose.

If foods cause hives, you have options available. Lamb and rice almost never cause allergic reactions. You can have a diet of only lamb and rice until free of hives. Add foods to the diet one at a time and watch for hives. Doctors call this an elimination diet.

Itching may be relieved by cold compresses, acetaminophen (p. 149), or antihistamines such as diphenhydramine or chlorpheniramine (p. 146).

WHAT TO EXPECT

If you're having a severe reaction with difficulty breathing or other systemic symptoms, the doctor may give you a shot of adrenaline (epinephrine) and other drugs.

For the typical case of hives, the doctor may prescribe an antihistamine or give an adrenaline shot to relieve swelling and itching. He or she may also try to find out what is causing an allergic reaction and develop a home treatment.

HIVES

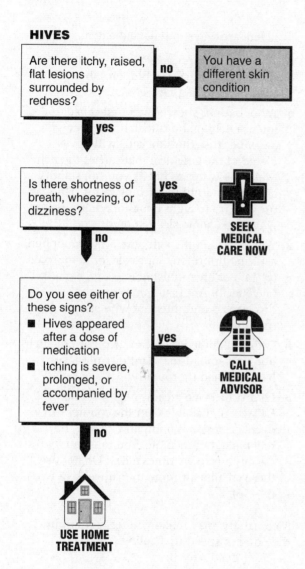

Are there itchy, raised, flat lesions surrounded by redness?

no → You have a different skin condition

yes ↓

Is there shortness of breath, wheezing, or dizziness?

yes → SEEK MEDICAL CARE NOW

no ↓

Do you see either of these signs?
- Hives appeared after a dose of medication
- Itching is severe, prolonged, or accompanied by fever

yes → CALL MEDICAL ADVISOR

no ↓

USE HOME TREATMENT

POISON IVY AND POISON OAK

Poison ivy and poison oak are plants containing oils that cause an allergic reaction of the skin. The first contact with their leaves sensitizes a person; later exposure will cause the formation of an itchy rash on the skin. The rash appears 12 to 48 hours after contact and lasts for up to two weeks.

Poison ivy and poison oak cause a rash of itchy, red blisters. The rash often appears as a line or welt where the plant brushed the skin.

You don't have to have direct contact with plants to get a skin reaction. Pets, contaminated clothing, or the smoke from burning plants can spread the oils.

HOME TREATMENT

Ideally you should learn to recognize these plants and avoid them. Once you have touched poison ivy or poison oak, remove the oils from your skin as soon as possible. Wash well with soap and water. Then wipe the skin with alcohol-soaked tissues or a washcloth wetted with rubbing alcohol to dissolve the oil. Rinse off. The solvent Tecnu can remove the oil as well. If you remove all the oil within six hours of exposure, you usually won't get the rash.

Scratching a rash caused by poison ivy or poison oak can lead to infection and delay healing. It's a good idea to trim your fingernails to avoid damaging the affected skin.

Here are ways to relieve the itch:

- Try a cool compress of Burow's solution (Domeboro, BurVeen, Bluboro) or an oatmeal bath (e.g., Aveeno).
- A hot bath or shower will first cause intense itching, but the itch will then go away because the skin cells will be depleted of the chemical that causes the itch. Make the water as hot as you can stand and stay in until the itching fades. This can provide up to eight hours of relief—a good way to get some sleep at night.
- You may treat the itch with acetaminophen, aspirin, ibuprofen, naproxen, or ketoprofen (p. 149) or an antihistamine (e.g., Benadryl or Vistaril). Antihistamines may cause drowsiness and interfere with sleep (p. 146).
- Plain calamine lotion can help with the itch but may spread the plant oil unless you have washed thoroughly.
- Hydrocortisone creams (e.g., Cortaid or Lanacort) available over the counter can decrease inflammation and itching, but relief is not immediate. You must apply the cream four to six times a day. Do not use these creams for more than a week or two (p. 156).

Medications may make you feel better but they do not speed up healing.

Call the doctor if:

- The rash is too large to treat at home
- Home treatment doesn't work
- Itching is intolerable
- The itchy areas are difficult to treat (e.g., around the eyes)

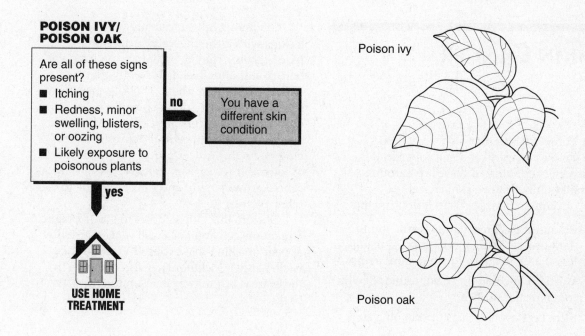

**POISON IVY/
POISON OAK**

Are all of these signs present?
- Itching
- Redness, minor swelling, blisters, or oozing
- Likely exposure to poisonous plants

no → You have a different skin condition

yes ↓

USE HOME TREATMENT

Poison ivy

Poison oak

WHAT TO EXPECT

The doctor will do a physical exam. He or she may prescribe a hydrocortisone cream stronger than you can buy over the counter. Or the doctor may give a steroid such as prednisone by mouth for a short time. The dose of oral steroids is large at first, then tapers off. Doctors usually give this only when a person has previously had a severe reaction to poison ivy or poison oak.

Skin Cancer

Nobody has perfect skin. Everybody has moles or warts or some superficial imperfection. Most of these are harmless. A small number can be skin cancer.

Common harmless skin lesions include:

- **Plain old freckles:** flat, uniform, tan to dark brown color, regular border, usually less than one-quarter inch (6 mm) across
- **Warts:** skin-colored, raised, rounded, with rough or flat surface
- **Skin tags:** wobbly tags of skin on a stalk
- **Seborrheic keratoses:** greasy, dirty tan to brown, raised, flat lesions; typically start to appear in mid-life on face, chest, and back; increase in number with age

Identifying skin cancer is not easy. When doctors aren't sure, they remove the lesion for testing. Most skin cancers fall into three categories.

Malignant melanoma is most common in people who have had one or more severe blistering sunburns before the age of 18. The most dangerous kind of skin cancer, malignant melanoma is sometimes described as moles that have changed. However, they are often flat, not raised like moles. Look for these warning signs:

- Changes in size, color, surface, shape, or border
- Variation in color—shades of red, white, and blue are warning signs
- An irregular border or edge

Squamous cell cancers are raised, bumpy lesions with a rough, scaly surface on a reddish base. They usually have an irregular border and often bleed. Typically they look like sores that don't heal. These lesions grow slowly and usually don't spread.

Basal cell cancers appear as pearly or waxy nodules with central depressions or craters. As this cancer grows, the center starts to look as if it has been gnawed. Basal cell cancer grows slowly and never spreads to other parts of the body.

Doctors link skin cancers to sun exposure. Squamous cell and basal cell cancers usually appear on skin most exposed to sun (head, neck, hands). Melanoma is also common in these areas but may appear on the chest or back.

HOME TREATMENT

Your best prevention strategy is to avoid sun exposure. Wear long sleeves, long pants, and hats with wide brims. Use a good sunscreen to prevent sunburn (p. 156).

You can do little for skin cancer but watch and wait. Examine your skin regularly and keep track of suspicious-looking spots. Have your doctor examine your skin during every physical exam.

WHAT TO EXPECT

A skin specialist (dermatologist) can usually give you the best advice about skin lesions. Usually the doctor can treat you on the first visit, often without surgery.

Once you have had skin cancer, you are likely to get it again. It is a good idea to have regular exams to make sure you have no new lesions. Avoid further sun damage to the skin.

SKIN CANCER

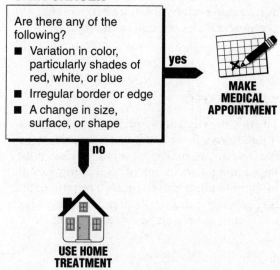

Are there any of the following?
- Variation in color, particularly shades of red, white, or blue
- Irregular border or edge
- A change in size, surface, or shape

yes → **MAKE MEDICAL APPOINTMENT**

no ↓

USE HOME TREATMENT

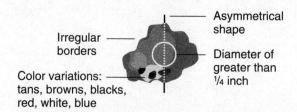

Asymmetrical shape

Irregular borders

Diameter of greater than ¼ inch

Color variations: tans, browns, blacks, red, white, blue

Characteristics of skin cancer. Look for changes in size, color, surface, or border. Tell the doctor about any questionable spots on your skin.

BOILS

A boil is a localized skin infection, usually due to staphylococcus bacteria. Boils may recur or persist for months, often affecting several family members at once.

Boils may be single or multiple, and can occur anywhere on the body. They range from pea-sized to the size of a walnut or larger.

Boils often begin as infections of the hair follicles. Other body parts prone to boils are areas under pressure, such as the buttocks. The infection begins beneath the skin and develops into an abscess, a pus-filled pocket. Eventually the abscess "points" toward the skin surface, ruptures, drains, and heals.

You should pay special attention to boils on the face. They are more likely to lead to serious infections.

HOME TREATMENT

The goal of treatment is to let out the pus, and to avoid pushing it deeper into the body. Avoid the temptation to squeeze the boil; handle all boils gently.

Apply warm, moist compresses to the area several times each day. Compresses help soften the skin for the rupture and drainage of a boil. Once a boil begins draining, the compresses will help keep the skin open. The more a boil drains, the better. An antibiotic ointment is optional; if used, don't let it prevent draining.

Frequent and thorough cleansing with soap and water will help prevent new infection. Some doctors like their patients to take antibiotics even though the boil is draining; a phone call (without a visit) to your doctor should be enough to find out about this.

WHAT TO EXPECT

The doctor will usually prescribe an antibiotic if you have a fever or a boil on the face.

The doctor may lance a boil if it has not yet drained. Lancing involves making a small incision to allow pus to drain. The pain of a boil eases as it drains. Although lancing a boil is a simple procedure, don't try it yourself.

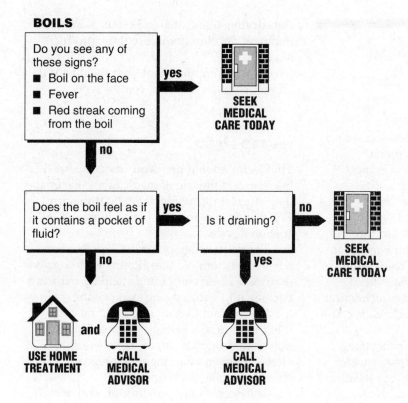

BOILS

Do you see any of these signs?
- Boil on the face
- Fever
- Red streak coming from the boil

yes → SEEK MEDICAL CARE TODAY

no ↓

Does the boil feel as if it contains a pocket of fluid?

yes → Is it draining? **no** → SEEK MEDICAL CARE TODAY

no ↓

USE HOME TREATMENT and CALL MEDICAL ADVISOR

yes ↓

CALL MEDICAL ADVISOR

ACNE

Acne is a disorder of the outermost skin layers, triggered by the hormonal changes of puberty. The condition is most common in teens with oily skin.

The acne pimple forms when hair follicles and skin glands become blocked with oil or plugs of keratin. Oil accumulates in the clogged pore, creating a place for bacteria to grow. Bacteria irritate the skin, resulting in pimples or sometimes larger cysts. (Blackheads are formed when air causes a chemical change of the keratin plugs. Blackheads cause minimal irritation.)

Contrary to popular belief, chocolate doesn't cause acne. Diet isn't a major factor in most cases. Still, avoid foods that seem to make your acne worse.

It is important not to scratch acne pimples. A pimple will disappear soon enough, but a scar caused by scratching will not.

HOME TREATMENT

Cleanse your skin several times a day. Scrubbing your face with a warm washcloth will help keep pores unplugged. Soap helps remove oil and bacteria on the skin. You can also use an abrasive soap (Pernox, Brasivol, etc.) one to three times daily. Steam can help unclog pores. Hot compresses are also sometimes helpful.

You should avoid cosmetic creams and greases, which can make acne worse. You may benefit from nonprescription remedies that contain benzoyl peroxide. You can also try a skin-drying agent such as Fostex. Skin irritation may develop if you use these products too often.

Make an appointment with the doctor if home treatment does not control acne.

WHAT TO EXPECT

The doctor should give you advice about skin hygiene and the use of medications. He or she may suggest ultraviolet (UV) light therapy. The doctor may remove blackheads with a suction device.

The doctor may prescribe a topical remedy such as retinoic acid (Retin-A) or benzoyl peroxide. These compounds help by reducing bacteria and encouraging skin peeling.

Isotretinoin (Accutane) is an oral drug that can help severe cases of acne. This is a powerful drug that can cause severe side effects. Women who might be pregnant should not take isotretinoin.

The doctor may prescribe an oral or topical antibiotic, or he or she may treat large, growing cysts with a corticosteroid shot.

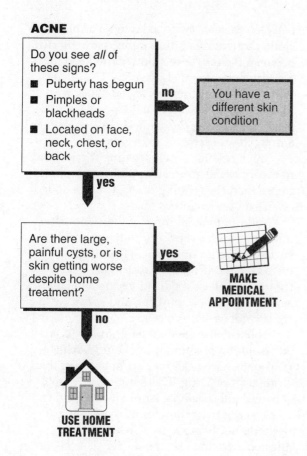

ACNE

Do you see *all* of these signs?
- ■ Puberty has begun
- ■ Pimples or blackheads
- ■ Located on face, neck, chest, or back

no → You have a different skin condition

yes ↓

Are there large, painful cysts, or is skin getting worse despite home treatment?

yes → **MAKE MEDICAL APPOINTMENT**

no ↓

USE HOME TREATMENT

FUNGAL INFECTIONS

Certain types of fungi can live happily on people's skin. Unfortunately, hosting these fungi does not make people happy.

Athlete's foot is the most common and persistent fungal infection. Itching toes are the major symptom. You might see redness and scaling between the toes, or even cracks and small blisters. Athlete's foot is very common during and after adolescence. Moisture is a major cause. Shared showers, baths, and locker rooms can spread the infection. Athlete's foot can be difficult to treat if it affects the toenails.

Jock itch is a fungal infection of the pubic region that primarily affects men. Friction and moisture make jock itch worse. Jock itch usually doesn't affect the scrotum or penis, and doesn't spread beyond the groin. The fungus gets its popular name from its ability to grow in an athletic supporter that's not laundered regularly.

Ringworm is a fungal infection that makes a characteristic red ring on the skin. The lesions start as small, red spots. When they grow to the size of a pea, the center begins to clear. At about the size of a dime, the lesions look like a ring. The spots often appear in groups that merge. In less common cases, ringworm affects the scalp or nails and is more difficult to treat.

HOME TREATMENT

You can often treat athlete's foot with scrupulous hygiene instead of medication. Wash between the toes twice a day with a soapy cloth. Dry your feet thoroughly, particularly between the toes. Use a powder to keep the feet dry, and put on clean socks. Use shoes that let your feet breathe. Avoid shoes with a plastic lining. Sandals or canvas sneakers are best. Not wearing the same shoes two days in a row allows each pair to dry out.

Treat jock itch by eliminating friction and moisture in the groin area. Wear boxer shorts rather than close-fitting briefs. Change soiled or sweaty underclothes often.

You can treat all three of these fungal infections with over-the-counter remedies such as Desenex, tolnaftate (Tinactin), miconazole (Micatin), or clotrimazole (Lotrimin). These medications are available as cream, solution, powder, and spray. Read the directions for proper use.

You can also treat athlete's foot with a 30% solution of aluminum chloride, which your pharmacist can prepare at less cost than a prescription drug. This solution dries the skin and kills bacteria. Apply it twice a day.

You can treat ringworm by applying Selsun Blue shampoo as a cream on the affected area, then letting it dry.

A fungal infection may take several weeks to resolve and often comes back. You should start seeing or feeling improvement after a week of home treatment. Call the doctor if the problem doesn't get better.

WHAT TO EXPECT

The doctor will take the history and do a physical exam. He or she may take skin scrapings for lab analysis, or examine the skin with an ultraviolet light (Wood's lamp).

If home treatment fails to control fungal infection, the doctor may prescribe haloprogin (Halotex) or ciclopirox (Loprox). Apply the cream or ointment as directed. The doctor may prescribe an oral drug, griseofulvin, for infection of the scalp or nails.

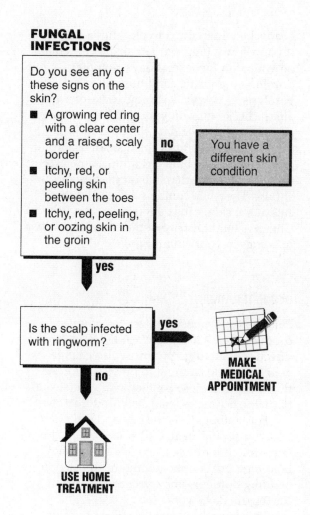

FUNGAL INFECTIONS

Do you see any of these signs on the skin?
- A growing red ring with a clear center and a raised, scaly border
- Itchy, red, or peeling skin between the toes
- Itchy, red, peeling, or oozing skin in the groin

no → You have a different skin condition

yes ↓

Is the scalp infected with ringworm?

yes → MAKE MEDICAL APPOINTMENT

no ↓

USE HOME TREATMENT

INSECT PROBLEMS

Our world is filled with lice and other tiny critters that have no respect for social status or income level. An itchy insect infestation does not reflect poorly on you or the cleanliness of your home.

Scabies is an irritation of the skin caused by a tiny mite. The mite easily spreads from person to person, or by contact with clothing and bedding. It burrows into the skin to lay eggs, leading to redness, swelling, and blisters. Often you can see its burrow as a red line, especially in a crease of skin. Scabies is very itchy. Scratching may obscure the burrows, and may result in infection.

Lice are hard to see without a magnifying glass. You may see clusters of eggs (nits) that look like tiny white clumps on hair strands. A louse bite leaves a small red spot that is very itchy. Although pubic lice ("crabs") can be spread during sexual contact, they aren't a venereal disease; toilet seats, infected linen, and other sources may spread them. Lice like to be close to a warm body all the time. They won't stay for long in clothing, bedding, or other places.

Bedbugs, like lice, live by sucking blood. They feed almost entirely at night because that's when you're in bed. Bedbugs strongly dislike light. The bite of the bedbug leaves a firm bump, usually clustered in twos and threes. People can develop allergies to bedbug bites, leading to severe itching and blisters.

Ticks are about one-quarter inch (6 mm) long—easy to see. In many areas ticks carry diseases, such as Rocky Mountain spotted fever and Lyme disease (p. 65). Call the doctor if you develop a fever, rash, joint pain, or headache within three weeks after a tick bite. If you allow a pregnant female tick to remain on your skin for several days, you may develop an unusual condition called tick paralysis. If you walk through tick-infested areas, check yourself, your children, and your pets several times a day.

Chiggers, like ticks, are a small hazard of nature. They are small red mites, sometimes called "redbugs," that live on grasses and shrubs. Their bite contains a chemical that eats at the skin, causing a tremendous itch. Chiggers tend to strike at the belt line or other openings in your clothing.

HOME TREATMENT

For lice, you can use an over-the-counter product (e.g., A200, Cuprex, RID). Read the directions carefully. You must also change your linen and clothing to prevent reinfestation. People in close contact with you (sexual partners, bedmates, etc.) also need treatment.

For bedbugs, it is the bed and the room that you should treat. Call your local health department for help. Chemical sprays may be useful, but simply getting the infested bedding outdoors and exposed to sun and air for several days works too.

You should remove ticks from the skin, although they will eventually fall off. The trick is to get the tick to let go; healing may take longer if mouth parts remain in your skin. Don't squeeze the tick, as that might raise your risk of diseases. With tweezers or gloved fingers, grasp the tick as close to the skin as possible; pull straight out with slow, even pressure. If the head is left under the skin, soak gently with warm water twice daily until healing is complete. If there is a red area around the bite more than two inches (5 cm) across, see the doctor.

INSECT PROBLEMS

Do you see any of these signs?

- An itchy line of raised red skin (scabies)
- Small white insects on the skin (lice)
- White lumps on hair shafts (lice nits)
- Bedbugs on or near the bed
- A tick stuck in or on the skin
- Itchy red sores around the beltline (chiggers)
- Itchy red sores after walking in grass near shrubs (chiggers)
- Small red mites on the skin, or a red spot in center of sore (chiggers)

no → You have a different skin condition

yes ↓

Is there a red area 2 inches (5 cm) across around a tick bite?

yes → **CALL MEDICAL ADVISOR**

no ↓

USE HOME TREATMENT

Nonprescription benzyl benzoate (25% solution) is effective against scabies but can be hard to find. Apply it once to the entire body except the face and around the opening of the penis or the vaginal opening. Wash it off 24 hours later. This medicine has an odor that some people find unpleasant. If you can't find benzyl benzoate, you'll have to get a prescription for lindane from your doctor.

Chiggers are better avoided than treated. Reduce your risk of chigger bites by using insect repellents, wearing appropriate clothing, and bathing after a visit to a chigger-infested area. Keep the bites clean. Soak them in warm water twice daily. Cuprex, RID, and A200 applied immediately may help kill the larvae, but the itch will persist.

For itching, we recommend cool soaks, calamine lotion, and/or pain relievers (p. 149). Antihistamines may help but often cause drowsiness (p. 146). You may try hydrocortisone creams (e.g., Cortaid, Lanacort), but they usually don't help much (p. 156). Don't use hydrocortisone products for long without talking to your doctor.

You should start feeling better within 72 hours of home treatment. Call the doctor if your symptoms last longer. It may take a while for your skin to return to normal.

WHAT TO EXPECT

The doctor will examine the entire skin surface to figure out the nature of the problem. He or she may use a magnifying glass, or take a scraping of the skin for laboratory analysis.

The doctor may prescribe lindane (e.g., Kwell, Scabene) for lice and chiggers. If a tick has bitten you, the doctor can remove the tick but can't prevent any disease that the tick might have transmitted. He or she may prescribe antibiotics.

CHILDHOOD DISEASES

Children are so prone to certain illnesses—chicken pox, mumps, and so on—that doctors have come to call these "childhood diseases." Fortunately, children recover from these diseases more readily than adults, and modern treatments have removed much of the danger. With vaccines, many people will never have these diseases at all.

Chicken Pox

The hallmark of chicken pox is an intensely itchy rash. Signs and symptoms appear 14 to 17 days after exposure to the chicken pox virus. The first sign of disease may be fatigue or fever 24 hours before the rash.

The rash goes through typical stages:

- It appears as flat red blotches, which grow into small pimples.

- The pimples grow into small, fragile blisters that look like drops of water on a red base. They typically appear in crops, first on the scalp and head, then all over the body. The blisters are most numerous over the shoulders, chest, and back.

- As the blisters break, the sores form a crust and start to itch intensely. Scratching may lead to infection of the sores, which could result in scars. Any fever usually subsides at this point.

- The crust falls away after nine to 13 days.

Chicken pox is very contagious. The virus can be transmitted from 24 hours before the rash until six days afterward. The virus spreads very easily through droplets from the mouth or through contact with contaminated articles of clothing. If one child has it, more than 90% of the time his or her siblings catch it.

Complications of chicken pox are rare. Very rarely, the virus can infect the brain (encephalitis). Infected sores require medical attention.

Usually having chicken pox gives you lifelong immunity. However, the virus remains in the body and can reappear as shingles (herpes zoster).

SHINGLES

The same herpes virus that causes chicken pox also causes shingles, and the individual who has had chicken pox may develop shingles (herpes zoster) later in life. Shingles is usually limited to one side of the body in a broad stripe, representing the skin area of a single nerve. Because it is limited to the nerve in which the virus is living, there is seldom fever, although there may be pain. Follow the same treatment as you do for chicken pox.

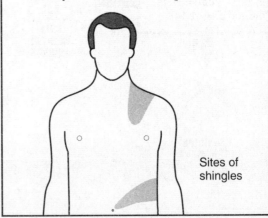

Sites of shingles

Measles

Measles is a highly contagious viral illness. The measles virus is spread by air and contact with contaminated clothing or other articles. It is a preventable disease that can be quite severe, so there is no excuse for not being vaccinated.

Symptoms begin about eight to 12 days after exposure to the virus:

■ Measles begins with fever, weakness, a dry, "brassy" cough, and inflamed eyes that are itchy, red, and sensitive to light.

■ Three to five days later, a pink, blotchy rash appears around the hairline, on the face, on the neck, and behind the ears. The spots darken and merge into red patches.

■ The rash spreads from head to chest to abdomen, and finally to the arms and legs. It may be mildly itchy, and lasts from four to seven days.

The person with measles is contagious from three to six days before the rash to several days afterward. Once you have had measles, or your measles vaccination, doctors consider you immune for life.

Complications of measles include sore throat, ear infections, and pneumonia. Very rarely, the person with measles may have a problem with blood clotting; this usually appears as dark purple splotches in the skin. Another rare but very serious complication is viral infection of the brain (encephalitis).

Mumps

Mumps is a viral infection of the salivary gland in the cheek in front of the ear. Signs and symptoms develop 16 to 18 days after exposure to the virus. You may have a low fever, headache, earache, or weakness. The fever can vary from only slightly above normal to as high as 104°F (40°C).

After several days, one or both salivary glands may swell. About a third of people with mumps show no swelling. When both sides swell, the person starts to look like a chipmunk! The mumps virus may affect other salivary glands, including those under the jaw and tongue.

Mumps is very contagious from two days before the first symptoms to the complete disappearance of swelling, usually about a week after it appears.

In children, mumps is generally a mild illness. Chewing and swallowing may be painful. Sour foods such as orange juice and pickles may make the pain worse.

Complications of mumps are more common in adults than in children, but still rare. They include viral infection of the brain (encephalitis), viral infection of the pancreas, kidney disease, and deafness. If the virus affects both testes or ovaries, mumps can result in sterility.

Rubella

Also known as German measles, rubella is a mild viral infection. It is less serious and less contagious than measles or chicken pox.

Rubella spreads from person to person by air. A person exposed to rubella may develop the disease 12 to 21 days later:

■ Symptoms may start with mild fatigue or enlarged lymph nodes at the back of the neck.

■ The person may develop a rash that first appears on the face, then quickly spreads to the trunk and limbs. The rash consists of clusters of flat or slightly raised red spots that merge into large patches. But the rubella rash can vary widely, and many people have no rash.

■ The person may have a fever up to 101°F (38°C) lasting two days or less.

About 10 to 15% of older children and adults with rubella feel joint pain. The pain usually begins on the third day of illness and can last until five days after the rash appears.

Complications of rubella are extremely rare. The main risk is to an unborn child. If a pregnant woman is exposed to rubella, the baby has an increased risk of birth defects: cataracts, heart disease, deafness, or mental retardation.

HOME TREATMENT

You can give the child acetaminophen, ibuprofen, naproxen, or ketoprofen to reduce pain and lower fever (p. 149). Because of the risk of Reye's syndrome, never give aspirin to children or teenagers who may have a viral infection, such as a cold, influenza, or chicken pox.

The main problems of chicken pox are fever and intense itching. To relieve the itch:

- Antihistamines may help (p. 146).
- Warm baths with oatmeal (e.g., Aveeno) or baking soda (one-half cup to a tubful of water) often help.
- For lesions in the mouth, gargling with salt water may give comfort: add one-half teaspoon (3 ml) salt to an eight-ounce (150 ml) glass of water.
- Scratching can cause bacterial infection. Wash an infected child's hands three times a day. Cut his or her fingernails. You can also put gloves on the child's hands. Finally, wash the whole skin gently but thoroughly each day.

Call the doctor if bacterial infection becomes severe and results in fever, if you can't control itching, or if the problem lasts more than three weeks.

A child with measles should be isolated until he or she is no longer contagious. Anybody in contact with the child who has not had measles should be vaccinated immediately. The child may feel generally sick or "measley," and be more comfortable if the room is dimly lit. You can use a vaporizer if the child has a cough.

The child with mumps may have difficulty swallowing, but it's important that he or she drink enough fluids. Avoid sour foods, such as orange juice. Adults who have never had mumps should avoid exposure to the child until the swelling resolves. Call the doctor if swelling hasn't gone down within three weeks.

You don't need to isolate the child with rubella, except from women who could be pregnant. They should avoid all exposure to the disease. Rubella usually requires no home therapy.

WHAT TO EXPECT

Don't be surprised if the doctor treats these diseases over the phone. Usually, seeing the doctor isn't necessary unless you have complications. Exposing others to infectious disease isn't wise—chicken pox is a minor illness to healthy kids, but can be fatal to others with medical problems.

If you see the doctor, he or she will take a history and do a physical examination. The doctor may run blood tests. If the person has signs that could suggest encephalitis, the doctor may do a spinal tap to obtain a sample of spinal fluid for laboratory analysis. The person may need to stay in the hospital.

There are no drugs to cure these illnesses or kill the viruses. The doctor may suggest

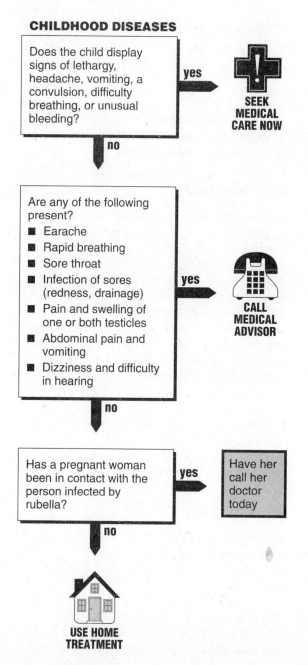

CHILDHOOD DISEASES

Does the child display signs of lethargy, headache, vomiting, a convulsion, difficulty breathing, or unusual bleeding?

yes → SEEK MEDICAL CARE NOW

no

Are any of the following present?
- Earache
- Rapid breathing
- Sore throat
- Infection of sores (redness, drainage)
- Pain and swelling of one or both testicles
- Abdominal pain and vomiting
- Dizziness and difficulty in hearing

yes → CALL MEDICAL ADVISOR

no

Has a pregnant woman been in contact with the person infected by rubella?

yes → Have her call her doctor today

no

USE HOME TREATMENT

supportive measures while the disease runs its course. If you have a bacterial infection, the doctor will prescribe antibiotics.

Call your doctor if a pregnant woman may have been exposed to a person with rubella. The doctor can run a blood test to see if the woman is immune to rubella or could have problems with the pregnancy.

Doctors can prevent many viral diseases with vaccines. Talk to your doctor to make sure your immunizations are current.

ARTHRITIS

Arthritis means joints that are painful to move. They may be red, warm, or swollen as well. Many people use the "arthritis" label for pain that is really in muscle, tendon, ligament, or bone; we discuss this sort of musculoskeletal pain on page 66.

There are more than a hundred types of arthritis. The most common:

- Osteoarthritis can cause knobby swelling of finger joints. More seriously, it can affect knees, hips, neck, or spine. Some osteoarthritis happens to almost everyone in later life but is usually not too serious.

- Rheumatoid arthritis can cause you to feel sick and stiff all over, in addition to causing joint problems. It usually starts in mid-life.

- Gout mostly affects men. It causes severe attacks of pain and swelling in one joint at a time, often the big toe, ankle, or knee.

- Ankylosing spondylitis affects the back. It causes chronic sore back and morning stiffness. A person with ankylosing spondylitis may be unable to touch the toes.

The complications of arthritis usually develop slowly. You can prevent these problems more easily than you can correct them, so you should manage the condition correctly and carefully.

When to See the Doctor

Few people with arthritis need to see a doctor right away. Urgent problems are:

- Infection
- Nerve damage
- Fractures near a joint
- Gout

The first three could result in serious joint damage. Gout can be so painful that the victim needs immediate help.

HOME TREATMENT

You can reduce pain and swelling in the joints by taking aspirin, ibuprofen, naproxen, or ketoprofen (p. 149). Although acetaminophen can relieve pain it doesn't reduce inflammation, so doctors seldom use it to treat arthritis other than osteoarthritis. Stomach irritation is the major concern. Ibuprofen and naproxen are less likely to cause stomach problems than aspirin but are more expensive. The signs of too much aspirin include ringing ears, dizziness, and hearing problems.

Resting an inflamed joint can speed healing. Heat can also help. Working a painful joint through its range of motion twice a day will help prevent stiffness.

If pain, swelling, or stiffness persists for six weeks, see a doctor.

WHAT TO EXPECT

The doctor will examine the joints and may have blood tests and X-rays done. He or she may use a needle to sample fluid from an affected joint.

The doctor may prescribe a nonsteroidal anti-inflammatory drug (NSAID), such as Feldene or Voltaren. Their effects, both good and bad, are very similar to aspirin, ibuprofen, or naproxen. Lower the risk of upset stomach by taking the tablets after meals or with an antacid.

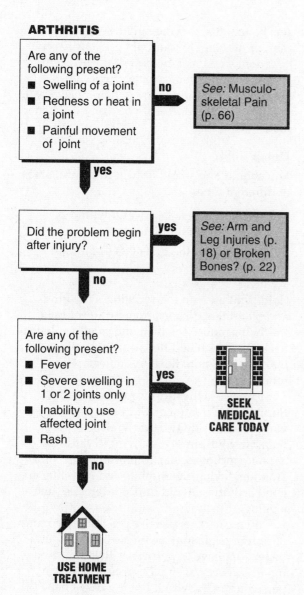

ARTHRITIS

Are any of the following present?
- Swelling of a joint
- Redness or heat in a joint
- Painful movement of joint

no → *See:* Musculo-skeletal Pain (p. 66)

yes ↓

Did the problem begin after injury?

yes → *See:* Arm and Leg Injuries (p. 18) or Broken Bones? (p. 22)

no ↓

Are any of the following present?
- Fever
- Severe swelling in 1 or 2 joints only
- Inability to use affected joint
- Rash

yes → **SEEK MEDICAL CARE TODAY**

no ↓

USE HOME TREATMENT

Corticosteroid drugs such as prednisone can reduce inflammation, but cause serious side effects after long-term use. Talk to your doctor if you take them for more than a few weeks. The doctor may inject corticosteroid drug into a painful joint. This usually shouldn't be done more than three times.

Rheumatoid arthritis may require stronger drugs such as methotrexate, gold salts, or hydroxychloroquine. Patients should be seen early by a specialist (rheumatologist), and should have periodic follow-ups.

LYME DISEASE

Lyme disease is an infection spread by ticks, usually the deer tick. An oval "bull's-eye" skin rash is a distinctive sign of the infection. The rash appears three to 20 days after the bite of an infected tick. The person with Lyme disease may also have fever, headache, stiff neck, and backache. Some people with the illness then develop arthritis within one to 22 weeks. A few get heart or neurological problems. Call your doctor if you see the "bull's-eye" rash on your skin. (See "Insect Problems," page 58.)

MUSCULOSKELETAL PAIN

Pain in a muscle or joint with no swelling or redness can be caused by tension, viral infection, or unusual physical activity. Sometimes joint or muscle pain has no obvious cause. These pains aren't arthritis, and they rarely suggest a serious disease. Muscle or joint pain usually goes away by itself.

Muscle or joint pain may be caused by thyroid disease, cancer, polymyositis (inflammation of the muscles), or polymyalgia rheumatica (aching in the neck, shoulder, and hip muscles that can affect the elderly). Pain at the upper neck and base of the skull is usually minor.

Fibromyalgia is marked by muscle pain, fatigue, and difficulty getting restful sleep. The person with fibromyalgia may also have irritable bowel syndrome, morning stiffness, anxiety, memory loss, and other symptoms.

Make an appointment if you have fever, weight loss, or severe fatigue. Otherwise, try home treatment for several weeks.

HOME TREATMENT

Rest and exercise and good sleep habits are important for musculoskeletal disorders. A program of slowly increasing exercise can help restore muscle tone. Walking, bicycling, and swimming are good activities. Use warm baths, massage, and stretching exercises as often as possible.

Poor work habits are a common cause of muscle and joint pain. If you work on hard floors, try sponge-soled shoes. A better chair may help if you work at a desk. Many people feel better after a change in lifestyle, switching jobs, or moving. If your pain goes away on vacation, stress may be part of the problem.

Acetaminophen, aspirin, ibuprofen, naproxen, or ketoprofen may help relieve pain (p. 149). Call the doctor if you don't feel better after three weeks.

Hot or Cold?

You should apply cold or heat to painful areas at different times:

- Use cold for new injury and within 24 hours of the first inflammation.
- Use heat after the first stages of inflammation.

Cold right after an injury reduces the fluid and blood that escape into joints or muscle; this helps reduce the pain and swelling. Later, heat increases blood flow during healing, makes joints more flexible, and can relieve muscle spasm.

Exercise is the most important part of fibromyalgia treatment. Start and increase your exercise slowly. Stretch for flexibility. Increase your physical activity toward full aerobic cardiovascular conditioning (p. 132). Walking, hiking, swimming, and bicycling are good activities. Avoid impact exercises such as jogging or tennis.

If you start an exercise program, the pain of fibromyalgia may be worse before it gets better. You have to persevere. Relief may be months away. Varying degrees of pain can persist for many years. But it will get better.

If you are not feeling better within two weeks, see your doctor.

WHAT TO EXPECT

The doctor will do a physical exam and request blood tests. He or she will probably

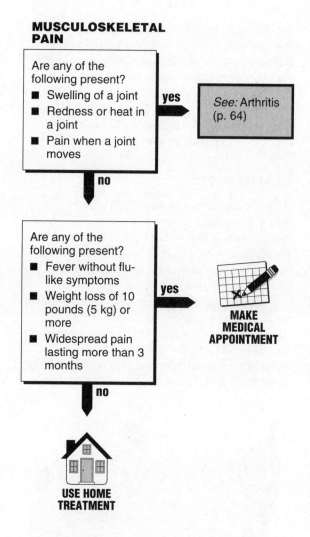

MUSCULOSKELETAL PAIN

Are any of the following present?

- Swelling of a joint
- Redness or heat in a joint
- Pain when a joint moves

yes → *See:* Arthritis (p. 64)

no

Are any of the following present?

- Fever without flu-like symptoms
- Weight loss of 10 pounds (5 kg) or more
- Widespread pain lasting more than 3 months

yes → **MAKE MEDICAL APPOINTMENT**

no

USE HOME TREATMENT

give advice similar to the home treatment described above.

If a specific joint in the body is causing the pain, a corticosteroid shot may help.

The doctor may manage fibromyalgia with drug regimens such as amitriptyline (Elavil) an hour or so before bedtime and an antidepressant (e.g., Prozac) in the morning. The goal of medication is to improve sleep without causing drowsiness during the day.

NECK PAIN

Most neck pain, such as the common "stiff neck," is due to muscle strain or spasm. You can care for this kind of minor pain at home.

Neck pain can be part of a flu syndrome that includes fever, headache, and muscle aches. If the person with neck pain also has general muscle aches, a visit to a doctor probably won't help.

Causes of neck pain that require a doctor's attention are:

- **Meningitis** Neck pain accompanied by fever and headache (but without general muscle aches) can signal this serious inflammation of the brain covering. With a very stiff neck, the person with meningitis may be unable to touch the chin to the chest. If you aren't sure, you're better off seeing the doctor for an ordinary muscle spasm than ignoring this **emergency** sign.

- **Pinched Nerve** Arthritis or neck injury can result in a pinched nerve. You may feel pain running down one arm, or numbness or tingling in one arm or hand. The symptoms appear on only one side, and neck stiffness is not the main complaint.

HOME TREATMENT

Morning neck pain may be due to poor sleeping habits. Sleep on a firm mattress; a bed board will make a mattress firmer. Stop using a pillow or use special pillows that keep the head from twisting.

Warmth may help spasms and pain. You can use hot showers, hot compresses, or a heating pad. Be careful with heat—skin burns easily. Aspirin, ibuprofen, or naproxen will help relieve pain and inflammation (p. 149).

Neck pain is slow to improve and may take several weeks to resolve. Call the doctor if you aren't better in a week.

WHAT TO EXPECT

If the doctor suspects meningitis, he or she will do a spinal tap and blood tests. You may have X-rays taken of the neck. The doctor may prescribe a neck collar. If he or she suspects nerve damage, the doctor may refer you to a neurologist or neurosurgeon.

The doctor may prescribe a muscle relaxer and perhaps a pain reliever. Prescription drugs aren't necessarily better than over-the-counter pain relievers. If you don't have infection or nerve damage, you're usually just as well off with home treatment.

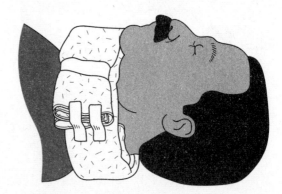

Bedtime neck pain relief. An ordinary bath towel can relieve neck pain. Before going to bed, fold a bath towel into a long strip four inches (10 cm) wide. Wrap it around the neck and secure it with tape or a safety pin. A soft neck collar from the drugstore works the same way. You usually will not need to wear the towel or collar during the day.

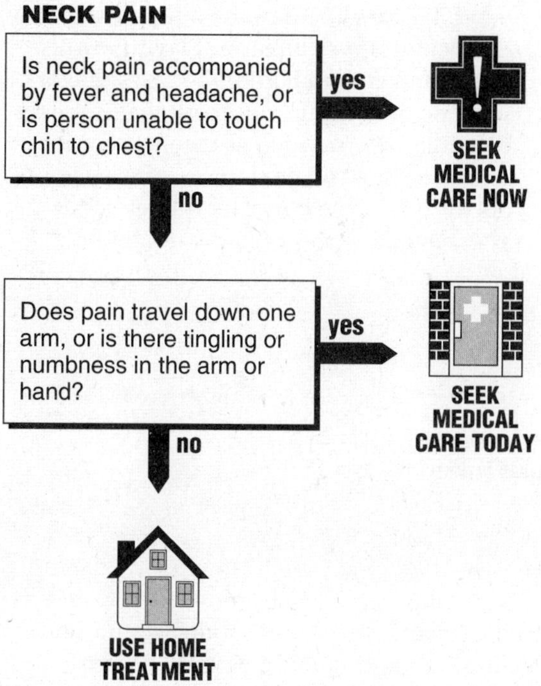

NECK PAIN

Is neck pain accompanied by fever and headache, or is person unable to touch chin to chest?

yes →

SEEK MEDICAL CARE NOW

no ↓

Does pain travel down one arm, or is there tingling or numbness in the arm or hand?

yes →

SEEK MEDICAL CARE TODAY

no ↓

USE HOME TREATMENT

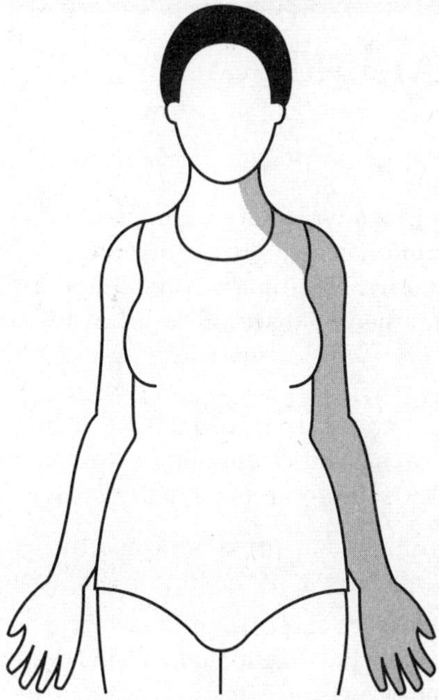

Sites of pinched nerve pain

ARM PAIN

Pain in the wrist, elbow, or shoulder is common and rarely serious. One exception is pain down the inner part of either arm, accompanied by discomfort just inside the breast bone; this could be the sign of a heart attack (p. 85).

The wrist is an unusual joint. A stiff wrist rarely causes difficulties, but a wobbly wrist does. Wrist pain can have many causes:

- Rheumatoid arthritis or osteoarthritis, especially pain in the thumb side (p. 64).

- If you have fever or rapid swelling as well, you may have an infection. This requires prompt medical attention.

- In carpal tunnel syndrome, a nerve is squeezed as it passes through the wrist. Your fingers may feel numb or pain may shoot down the fingers or up the forearm. The finger numbness doesn't affect the little finger, and usually doesn't involve the outer half of the ring finger. If you tap the inner wrist, you may get a sudden tingling in the fingers similar to hitting your funny bone. The tingling and pain may be worse at night or when you flex your wrists.

Elbow pain, if it does not follow an injury, usually has one of these causes:

- **Bursitis** The elbow bursa is a fluid-filled sac at the tip of the elbow. When irritated, the bursa can swell to the size of a small egg. The swelling is painful but does not cause fever or redness.

- **Tennis elbow** This condition occurs after repeated twisting of the forearm, wrist, and hand. It causes pain in the outer area of the elbow and upper forearm. Playing tennis causes fewer than half of the cases doctors see. The rest result from work that involves twisting the arm, such as using a screwdriver, or have no obvious cause. See your doctor if tennis elbow doesn't get better after several weeks of home treatment.

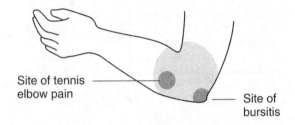

Site of tennis elbow pain

Site of bursitis

Shoulder pain comes most often from soft tissue (ligaments, tendons, bursae) and not from the shoulder bones or joint. Because doctors treat common shoulder pains the same, you need not worry about which condition you have. However, these signs indicate a more serious problem:

- Arm injuries (p. 18) in connection with shoulder pain

- Fever, swelling, and redness—see the doctor about possible infection

- Inability to move the arm—see the doctor

If in doubt about a shoulder pain, call your doctor.

HOME TREATMENT

Splinting is the key to managing wrist pain. Wrist splints are available at medical supply stores and many drug stores. Wear the splint all the time for a few days, then just at night for a few weeks. If the problem persists after six weeks of home treatment, see the doctor.

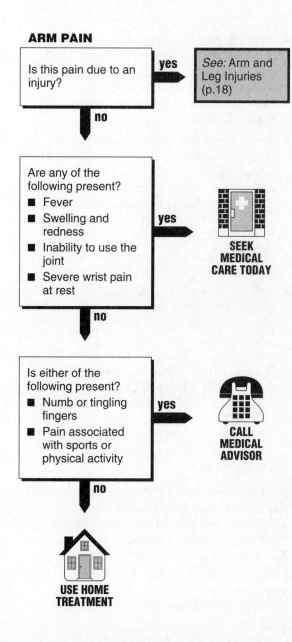

ARM PAIN

Is this pain due to an injury? — **yes** → *See:* Arm and Leg Injuries (p.18)

no ↓

Are any of the following present?
- Fever
- Swelling and redness
- Inability to use the joint
- Severe wrist pain at rest

— **yes** → **SEEK MEDICAL CARE TODAY**

no ↓

Is either of the following present?
- Numb or tingling fingers
- Pain associated with sports or physical activity

— **yes** → **CALL MEDICAL ADVISOR**

no ↓

USE HOME TREATMENT

For painful bursae and tendons, the key word is RIMS:

- **Rest** At the first sign of discomfort, cut down on your activity. Warm up slowly and stretch before exercise.

- **Ice** At the first pain, apply ice for 30 minutes, then let the hurt joint rewarm for 15 minutes. Continue this cycle for one to two hours. Be careful not to freeze the skin.

- **Mobility** Rest the arm for 24 to 48 hours. Then, gently put your arm through range of motion exercise several times a day.

- **Strengthening** Start gradual exercise to strengthen the arm muscles. We recommend use of ice afterward. Wait three to six weeks before returning to the activity that caused the problem.

You may take acetaminophen or other pain reliever as needed. Call a doctor if the condition persists beyond three weeks.

WHAT TO EXPECT

The doctor will examine the arm. He or she may request X-rays of the affected area, but this is rare. The doctor may give a corticosteroid injection. He or she should give such injections only if home therapy doesn't work. The doctor should give no more than two or three such injections.

The doctor may prescribe nonsteroidal anti-inflammatory drugs (NSAIDs). Similar to aspirin, these drugs decrease pain but don't speed the healing process.

The doctor should instruct you in rehabilitation exercises.

Surgery is an option for several conditions. The doctor may treat rheumatoid arthritis and carpal tunnel nerve syndrome surgically. Surgery is the last resort and is a gamble; satisfaction isn't guaranteed.

LOW BACK PAIN

Low back pain is frustrating for doctors and patients alike. It's slow to heal and often comes back.

The cause of low back pain is usually an injury to the ligaments or other tissue, though it can be a herniated disk. The pain can be severe or moderate, or you can simply feel stiff. The pain is usually felt in the back, sometimes in the buttocks or upper leg as well.

Often the cause isn't clear. The pain may start immediately after a muscle strain, or hours later. Severe pain usually lasts for 48 to 72 hours, followed by days or weeks of less severe pain.

Back pain that results from a severe blow or fall may require immediate attention.

Back pain may extend down the leg *below the knee* if a sciatic nerve is pinched. Doctors call this sciatica. This pain often responds to home treatment. Signs that you should see the doctor right away for sciatica include:

- Loss of bladder or bowel control
- Weakness in the leg

HOME TREATMENT

The low back pain syndrome is a vicious cycle: injury causes the pain of muscle spasm, and the spasm leads to more pain. To heal most rapidly, you must avoid reinjury and allow your back to recover.

- Avoid reinjury by limiting your physical activity. If necessary, rest flat on your back for the first 24 hours.

- After the first day, moderate activity—as much as the pain allows—is better than bed rest. Strenuous activity during the next six weeks can make the problem worse, however. After recovery, an exercise program will help prevent reinjury.

- If you suffer from low back pain, sleep without a pillow on a very firm mattress, a waterbed, or even the floor. A bed board under your mattress will make it firmer. You may find it more comfortable to sleep with a towel folded under the small of your back or a pillow beneath your knees.

- A heat pack applied to the back will help relieve pain.

- You can take acetaminophen, aspirin, ibuprofen, naproxen, or ketoprofen (p. 149).

If there is no nerve damage, you don't gain anything by going to the doctor for low back pain. Being careful and easing the symptoms will help your back recover. If severe back pain lasts more than a week, call the doctor.

WHAT TO EXPECT

The doctor will ask questions and do a physical exam to look for causes of back pain. X-rays may be taken of the back, particularly if the pain is due to a fall or blow. If the doctor suspects that nerves may have been hurt, you may have special imaging studies done, such as myelogram, computerized tomography (CT), or magnetic resonance imaging (MRI).

In rare cases, when nerves are at risk, the doctor may hospitalize the person. Treatment may include traction or surgery.

Usually the doctor gives advice similar to the home treatment we describe above. He or she may prescribe a muscle relaxant or a pain reliever. Back exercises, relaxation, and biofeedback may help chronic low back pain.

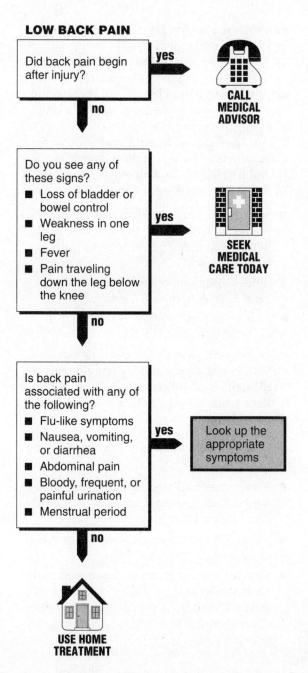

LOW BACK PAIN

Did back pain begin after injury?

yes → **CALL MEDICAL ADVISOR**

no ↓

Do you see any of these signs?
- Loss of bladder or bowel control
- Weakness in one leg
- Fever
- Pain traveling down the leg below the knee

yes → **SEEK MEDICAL CARE TODAY**

no ↓

Is back pain associated with any of the following?
- Flu-like symptoms
- Nausea, vomiting, or diarrhea
- Abdominal pain
- Bloody, frequent, or painful urination
- Menstrual period

yes → Look up the appropriate symptoms

no ↓

USE HOME TREATMENT

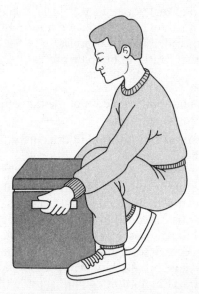

Lifting heavy objects. To avoid back strain, bend your knees but keep your back straight and erect.

HIP PAIN

Because the hip joint is so deep inside the body, identifying the source of hip pain can be difficult. An injury or disease of the hip may be felt in the groin, outer thigh, or down the leg to the knee. Pain felt in the hip may actually start in the lower back.

Although the hip is one of the body's strongest and best-protected joints, it is still subject to dislocation, fracture, and soft-tissue injury. The narrow neck of the thigh bone (femur) can break easily, particularly among elderly people who slip or fall. The artery to the end of that bone can get blocked, leading to the death of bone tissue and a form of arthritis called aseptic necrosis.

Other causes of hip pain are:

- Infection
- Bursitis—inflammation of the fluid-filled sacs over the joint
- Rheumatoid arthritis and osteoarthritis (p. 64)

A stiff hip may not be painful, but it can place extra strain on the lower back. The form of arthritis called ankylosing spondylitis can cause hip stiffness. Hip problems can lead to a flexion contracture, in which the hip joint becomes fixed in a slightly bent position, losing some range of motion.

HOME TREATMENT

Pay attention to pain. Avoid activities that make your hip worse. Rest the joint after painful activities. Avoid pain medication as much as possible.

Use a cane or crutches if needed. Hold the cane in the hand *opposite* the painful hip. This allows the large muscles around the sore hip joint to relax. Move the cane forward along with the affected hip.

As the hip pain lessens, gradually introduce exercise. Use gentle motion exercises at first to free the hip and reduce stiffness. Repeat these exercises two or three times a day:

- Stand with your good hip by a table. Lean on the table with your hand. Swing the leg with the bad hip from side to side and front and back.
- Spread your legs as far as you can and bend from side to side.
- With your legs together, turn your feet outward like a duck.
- Lie on your back on the edge of your bed with your bad hip and leg hanging just off the mattress. Stretch your leg toward the floor while keeping your knees as straight as you can.

Introduce more activity to strengthen the hip muscles:

- Lie on your back and raise your legs one at a time. Keep the leg straight and lift until you reach a 45° angle.
- Swim. This stretches muscles and builds good tone.
- Bicycle or walk. When walking, start with short strides and gradually lengthen them as you loosen up. Gradually increase your efforts and distance, but not by more than 10% each day.

A good, firm bed will help. The best sleeping position is on your back. Avoid

HIP PAIN

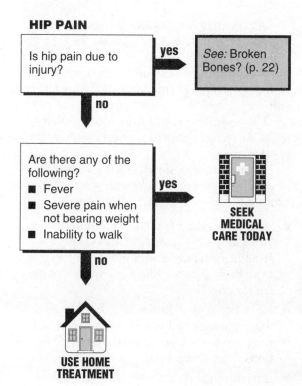

Is hip pain due to injury? **yes** → *See:* Broken Bones? (p. 22)

no ↓

Are there any of the following?
- Fever
- Severe pain when not bearing weight
- Inability to walk

yes → **SEEK MEDICAL CARE TODAY**

no ↓

USE HOME TREATMENT

pillows beneath the knees or under the lower back. Make sure you take anti-inflammatory medication as prescribed, especially if you have rheumatoid arthritis or ankylosing spondylitis.

If pain persists after six weeks of home treatment, see the doctor.

WHAT TO EXPECT

The doctor will examine the hip and its range of motion. You may have X-rays taken. The doctor may prescribe anti-inflammatory medication. Rarely, the doctor may give you a shot.

The doctor may recommend surgery if your pain is intense and persistent, or if you are having problems walking. Total hip replacement is usually successful. An artificial hip lasts at least ten to 15 years. You will be able to get up and around soon after surgery. Complications of surgery are rare.

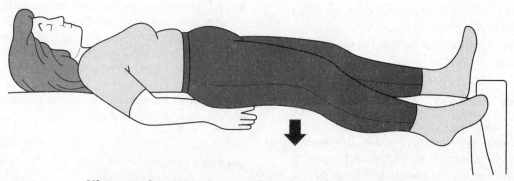

Hip exercise. With your shoulders, trunk, and one leg resting on the bed, allow the leg with the injured hip to dangle off the bed. Bend your knee as little as possible as you stretch the leg and hip backward, toward the floor.

KNEE PAIN

The knee is a large, strong joint, but it does not tolerate side stresses very well. The engineering of the knee makes it prone to both injury and degenerative disease. People are more likely to have these problems if they are overweight.

To work properly, the knee must bend and straighten while keeping stable support. The knee should not wobble from side to side. Make an appointment with the doctor if:

- Your knee is unstable or wobbles
- You cannot completely straighten or bend the knee

A knee that is red or feels hot may have an infection or gout. Pain or swelling in the calf below a sore knee suggest a blood clot or a cyst. See a doctor promptly if:

- You cannot walk
- Your knee is very painful even when it's not bearing weight
- You have pain or swelling in the calf or thigh

HOME TREATMENT

Pay attention to your pain. Avoid activities that make pain worse. You can take acetaminophen, aspirin, ibuprofen, naproxen, or ketoprofen to ease pain (p. 149), but don't use these medications to ignore what the pain is telling you.

If you have arthritis, make sure you take your medication as directed.

A cane may help reduce the stress on your knee. Most people use the cane on the *same* side as the painful knee.

Do not use a pillow under the knee while resting or sleeping. This can make your knee stiff.

Knee pain can result from foot problems; make sure your shoes fit properly and are in good shape.

Start exercising slowly. Increase your level of activity until you are exercising several times daily. Here is a gradual program:

- Start by bending and straightening the leg. Work at getting it straight and keeping it straight. You may find it more comfortable to sit or lie down while a friend moves the leg for you.

- Next, begin gentle exercises. Tighten your thigh muscles and hold for two seconds, then rest for two seconds. Do ten repetitions three times a day.

- Introduce gentle activity. A bicycle in low gear is a good place to start. Stationary bicycles are fine. Be sure that the seat is high enough so your knee doesn't bend to more than a right angle as you pedal.

- Swimming and walking are very good activities for knees. Gradually increase your distance. Avoid exercise and activities that involve deep knee bends; these place too much stress on the knee.

See your doctor if your knee is painful after six weeks of home treatment.

WHAT TO EXPECT

The doctor will examine your knee and other joints. You may have an X-ray done of your knee. The doctor may use a needle to draw fluid from the knee.

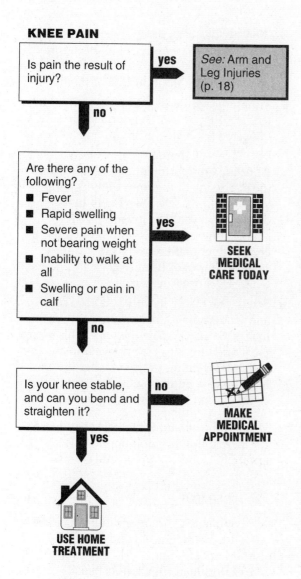

KNEE PAIN

Is pain the result of injury? — **yes** → *See:* Arm and Leg Injuries (p. 18)

no

Are there any of the following?
- Fever
- Rapid swelling
- Severe pain when not bearing weight
- Inability to walk at all
- Swelling or pain in calf

yes → **SEEK MEDICAL CARE TODAY**

no

Is your knee stable, and can you bend and straighten it? — **no** → **MAKE MEDICAL APPOINTMENT**

yes

USE HOME TREATMENT

Several operations are helpful for knee problems, including surgery to trim or remove cartilage. Increasingly, doctors are using an arthroscope to diagnose and treat knee problems. This is a minor procedure.

For severe and persistent problems, the doctor may suggest total knee replacement. This surgery is usually successful in giving total pain relief.

CRUTCHES

Crutches should be short enough that you don't injure the nerves in your armpits by leaning on the crutches. Take the weight on your hands or arms. When a person stands straight, crutches should reach from six inches to the side of the feet to two inches—or three to four fingers' width—below the armpits.

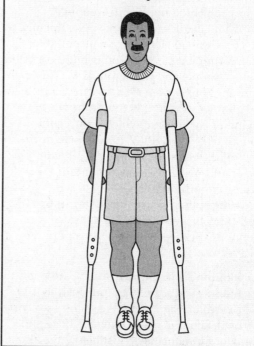

LEG PAIN

Leg pain that isn't caused by injury can often be traced to one of three conditions:

- **Thrombophlebitis:** inflammation and the formation of clots in leg veins
- **Intermittent claudication:** narrowing of leg arteries
- **Shin splints:** "overuse" injuries resulting from vigorous exercise

Thrombophlebitis is most likely after a period of prolonged rest, such as a long car or plane ride. It appears as a generalized ache, not starting from a specific point. You may feel warmth and a tender vein in the middle of the calf. Thrombophlebitis requires immediate medical attention so the doctor can detect any blood clots as soon as possible.

Intermittent claudication is more common in older people and heavy smokers. This pain is brought on by exercise and relieved by a few minutes of rest. It is caused by the narrowing of leg arteries, which reduces the amount of blood delivered to muscle during such mild exercise as walking. Call your doctor and make an appointment for the earliest opportunity.

"Shin splints" is a catch-all term for conditions that sometimes result from strenuous exercise, usually after a period of inactivity:

- **Posterior Tibial Shin Splints:** Pain and tenderness in a three- to four-inch (8–10 cm) area on the inner edge of the shin bone (tibia), about midway between knee and ankle. The bone itself, just below the skin, is not tender. This results from overstressing the tibia muscle where it attaches to the bone. It accounts for 75% of the pains athletes feel in the front portion of their legs.

- **Tibial Periostitis:** The tibial bone itself is tender. The pain and tenderness are similar to posterior tibial shin splints but are felt further toward the front of the leg.

- **Anterior Compartment Syndrome:** Pain on the outer side of the front of the leg that arises when muscles swell with blood during hard use. The muscle swelling squeezes blood vessels within the muscle compartment and reduces flow to the muscle. This pain usually goes away after ten to 15 minutes of rest.

- **Stress Fractures:** Sharply localized pain and tenderness in the tibia, one or two inches (3–5 cm) below the knee. This occurs most often two to three weeks into an increased training program, after the legs have taken a pounding. Stress fractures aren't treated with casts, but with rest.

Call your doctor for leg pain that doesn't fit the description of thrombophlebitis, intermittent claudication, or shin splints.

HOME TREATMENT

Thrombophlebitis and intermittent claudication need to be diagnosed and treated by a physician, not at home.

Posterior tibial shin splints usually respond to a week of rest, during which the tender area is iced twice a day for 20 minutes. Acetaminophen, aspirin, ibuprofen, naproxen, or ketoprofen with meals may help (p. 149). When the pain is gone, stretch the tibia muscles twice a day by extending the ankle joint so that the toes point down as far as possible. Consider an arch support if you

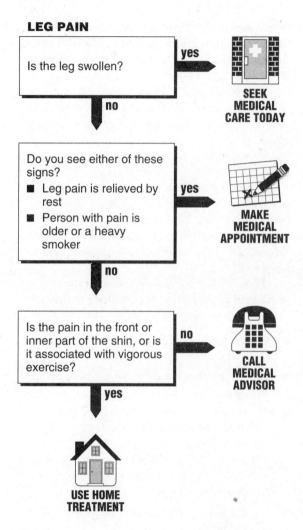

LEG PAIN

Is the leg swollen? — yes → **SEEK MEDICAL CARE TODAY**

no ↓

Do you see either of these signs?
- Leg pain is relieved by rest
- Person with pain is older or a heavy smoker

yes → **MAKE MEDICAL APPOINTMENT**

no ↓

Is the pain in the front or inner part of the shin, or is it associated with vigorous exercise? — no → **CALL MEDICAL ADVISOR**

yes ↓

USE HOME TREATMENT

have flat feet. Don't start running again for another two to four weeks, and then only at half speed, with a gradual increase in speed and distance.

Treat tibial periostitis the same as posterior tibial shin splints, except that you can gradually return to sports after one week of home care. Athletic shoes with good shock absorption, especially in the heel, are very important.

Anterior compartment syndrome almost always goes away as the muscle gets used to vigorous exercise. Rest for ten minutes when pain starts, then run slowly. Icing the leg for 20 minutes after running may help.

Stress fractures require rest from running, usually for a month, before starting to gradually recondition your legs. Complete healing takes four to six weeks. Crutches can be used but usually aren't necessary.

Call the doctor if you are unsure of the nature of your condition or have not improved after several weeks of home care.

WHAT TO EXPECT

A simple, painless test called impedance plethysmography (IPG) is very useful to detect thrombophlebitis in the thigh. If it is detected, the doctor may prescribe blood thinners (anticoagulants) to reduce the risk of a blood clot going to your lung. Anticoagulant therapy is not always effective and carries some risk of bleeding complications. Thrombophlebitis in the calf alone carries much less risk, so anticoagulant therapy may not be required. Regardless of testing and results, talk with your doctor about the therapy's risks and benefits before deciding.

Intermittent claudication is usually diagnosed by history and physical exam. In some cases, a special X-ray of the leg arteries (arteriogram) may be done. Treatment, if needed, includes surgical procedures to widen or bypass obstructed leg arteries.

Most shin splint injuries are cared for at home. In the rare case of compartment syndrome that doesn't improve, a simple surgical procedure can be done without a hospital stay to relieve the pressure in the muscle.

ANKLE PAIN AND SWELLING

Sprains and strains are the most common causes of ankle pain. The ligament stretching across the outer portion of the ankle is a frequent target for injury. An injured ankle may be painful and unstable, increasing the risk of further damage.

Arthritis can affect the bones and cartilage of the ankle. Arthritis can allow injured ligaments to slip and wobble, resulting in further stress, instability, and pain.

Swelling of the ankles without pain is usually due to an accumulation of fluid in the tissues (edema). Heart disease, lung disease, kidney disease, and liver disease can cause edema. Edema usually affects both legs. The swelling may involve the calves or thighs, but because of gravity edema is typically worse around the ankles. If you press your finger on a swollen area for a short time, you may leave behind a temporary indentation or pit.

If the swelling affects *only one leg* you may have a blood clot in a vein (thrombophlebitis). This swelling is usually rapid and painful. You may also see redness or feel warmth. Thrombophlebitis requires immediate medical attention.

HOME TREATMENT

Pay attention to pain. It is a signal of something wrong. If the ankle pain is due to injury, ease up on your exercise program and give your ankle more rest. You can use crutches or a cane to take weight off a hurt ankle.

High-lacing boots can give some support for an unstable ankle. Light hiking boots, which resemble running shoes that go above the ankle, often give excellent ankle support. A health professional can fit you for special ankle braces or boots.

If your painful ankle is stable, wear an elastic bandage (p. 155) and a comfortable shoe with a thick heel pad—jogging shoes are good.

If you have arthritis, take your medication as directed.

When the ankle pain eases, gently begin to exercise the joint again. Swimming is good because you don't have to bear weight. Start your exercises slowly and increase to several times daily. Take your time, be patient, and keep at it.

Therapy for edema depends on the underlying cause. The doctor will identify and treat that medical condition. In addition:

- A low-salt diet helps reduce fluid accumulation and ankle swelling.

- Exercise pushes fluid back into circulation and reduces swelling.

- Elevating your legs can help the fluid drain back into circulation. Recline with your legs raised higher than your heart. Place pillows or a folded blanket beneath your calves, not beneath your knees. Avoid sitting or standing for long periods.

- Avoid constricting clothing or garters. Wear support stockings.

WHAT TO EXPECT

The doctor will do an examination, paying particular attention to the circulation and the area around the ankles. If you injured your ankle the doctor may use X-rays to help in diagnosis. You may have blood tests done to evaluate kidney and liver function and to measure blood proteins.

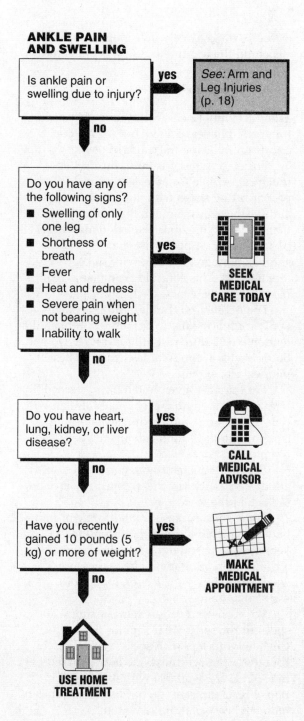

ANKLE PAIN AND SWELLING

Is ankle pain or swelling due to injury? — **yes** → *See:* Arm and Leg Injuries (p. 18)

no ↓

Do you have any of the following signs?
- Swelling of only one leg
- Shortness of breath
- Fever
- Heat and redness
- Severe pain when not bearing weight
- Inability to walk

yes → **SEEK MEDICAL CARE TODAY**

no ↓

Do you have heart, lung, kidney, or liver disease? — **yes** → **CALL MEDICAL ADVISOR**

no ↓

Have you recently gained 10 pounds (5 kg) or more of weight? — **yes** → **MAKE MEDICAL APPOINTMENT**

no ↓

USE HOME TREATMENT

Sometimes an ankle injury requires surgery to fuse ankle bones. A fixed ankle is far better than a painful, wobbly one.

The doctor may prescribe anti-inflammatory medications. He or she may also prescribe a splint, brace, crutches, or special shoes. With crutches, your hands and arms should bear your weight, not your armpits. When you stand straight:

- Each crutch tip should be six inches (15 cm) to the side of your foot.
- The crutches' tops should be two inches (5 cm) below your armpits.

With edema, treatment is based on its cause. The doctor may prescribe diuretics (water pills) that reduce body fluids by increasing urination. These drugs are effective, but they have side effects, such as causing you to lose potassium. Home treatment is generally better than medication.

FOOT PAIN

Several common soft-tissue injuries can cause tenderness and swelling in the foot.

- You can sprain a tendon in the foot (plantar fasciitis) or inflame the tendon along the back of the heel (Achilles tendinitis).

- Pressure from shoes can cause inflammation of the fluid-filled sac, or bursa, that surrounds the back of the heel (bursitis). Other bursae are under the heel. Landing hard or awkwardly on the heel can inflame these bursae.

- Tight-fitting shoes can squeeze feet, pinching nerves between the bones and causing a swelling called Morton's neuroma. Typically found between two bones in the middle of the foot, the swelling is very sensitive and can be intensely painful. You may also feel numbness between the toes.

- A bunion is an area of thickened skin on the inside of the foot resulting from the metatarsal bone rubbing against your shoe. The bunion can become inflamed and sore.

- Corns and calluses result from friction with ill-fitting shoes. Corns are lumps of thickened skin, usually found on the tops of toes. Calluses are less lumpy areas of thickened skin, and are more common on the ball of the foot.

- A virus causes plantar warts, which are found on the ball of the foot.

- Unaccustomed, heavy use of the feet, as in a sudden increase in running or basketball, may cause stress fractures. Pain usually comes on gradually. The long bone just behind the fourth toe is most vulnerable.

HOME TREATMENT

Take acetaminophen or another nonprescription pain reliever (p. 149), but focus your efforts on relieving the cause of pain.

For plantar fasciitis, rest your feet as much as possible for at least a week. Get proper-fitting shoes with good arch support and flexible soles. Tighten the laces a bit more than usual. A one-quarter-inch (6 mm) heel pad may help. A podiatrist or orthopedic surgeon may give you a device to keep the foot aligned. This condition can take a year or more to go away.

For Achilles tendinitis, stop exercising and apply ice twice daily to the tendon. Stretch the tendon well before resuming exercise. Do not bounce with a sore Achilles tendon. These injuries heal slowly.

For bursitis, seven to ten days' rest will help relieve the initial problem. Moleskin will relieve pressure on the skin. Get shoes stretched so they don't rub against your heel, or get new shoes.

For Morton's neuroma, wear shoes with enough room for your feet, especially around the ball of the foot.

For a bunion, use a small sponge or pad between the big toe and the second toe to keep the big toe straight. Moleskin or padding around the bunion may relieve pressure. Wear shoes that allow your feet enough room, especially the toes.

For corns and calluses, make sure your shoes fit properly. Wear sandals if you can. Cushion your feet with socks. Corn plasters containing salicylic acid (the active ingredient in aspirin) are available without a prescription. Use as directed; do not use other types of pain medication at the same time.

FOOT PAIN

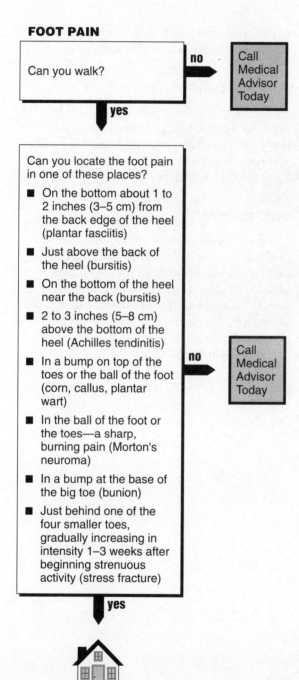

Can you walk? **no** → Call Medical Advisor Today

yes ↓

Can you locate the foot pain in one of these places?

- On the bottom about 1 to 2 inches (3–5 cm) from the back edge of the heel (plantar fasciitis)

- Just above the back of the heel (bursitis)

- On the bottom of the heel near the back (bursitis)

- 2 to 3 inches (5–8 cm) above the bottom of the heel (Achilles tendinitis)

- In a bump on top of the toes or the ball of the foot (corn, callus, plantar wart)

- In the ball of the foot or the toes—a sharp, burning pain (Morton's neuroma)

- In a bump at the base of the big toe (bunion)

- Just behind one of the four smaller toes, gradually increasing in intensity 1–3 weeks after beginning strenuous activity (stress fracture)

no → Call Medical Advisor Today

yes ↓

USE HOME TREATMENT

For plantar warts, use corn plasters and other nonprescription wart remedies. See the doctor if warts persist or get worse. Wear slippers or bath shoes to reduce the risk of spreading plantar warts.

For stress fractures, rest the foot. You may find crutches helpful for a week or so. A crack in a metatarsal may take six weeks to three months to heal.

WHAT TO EXPECT

For plantar fasciitis and bursitis, the doctor may give up to three cortisone shots if other therapy has failed. Surgery is a last resort.

The doctor may prescribe anti-inflammatory drugs for Achilles tendinitis. He or she may put a walking cast on the affected limb.

The doctor may give cortisone shots for Morton's neuroma if you have not obtained relief with oral medication and switching shoes. He or she may suggest you have the neuroma removed surgically, which usually leaves a region of skin on the foot permanently numb.

If you have an inflamed bunion, the doctor may give you a cortisone shot. If moleskin and shoe adjustments don't help, the doctor may recommend surgery to realign the big toe.

The doctor may use cold (liquid nitrogen), heat (electrocoagulation), or surgery to remove plantar warts. They often recur.

For metatarsal stress fractures, crutches will help keep weight off the affected foot. Doctors rarely splint these fractures with a cast, and almost never do surgery.

CHEST PAIN

Chest pain is a serious symptom meaning "heart attack" to most people. However, many things in the chest can cause pain. Often it's hard even for a doctor to figure out the cause.

There's no easy rule to decide which pains you may treat at home. If you have any doubts about chest pain, or have other symptoms such as shortness of breath, call 911 immediately.

The heart almost never causes pain for healthy men under 30 years of age or women under 40. Heart pain remains rare among men in their 40s and women in their 50s. Until middle age, chest pain is usually caused by something other than the heart:

- A brief, shooting pain is common in healthy young people and means nothing. So is a "catch" at the end of a deep breath.

- Hyperventilation is a common cause of chest pain, particularly in young people (p. 109).

- If you press at the spot of discomfort and cause or worsen the pain, it is probably coming from the chest wall, not the heart. You can treat this pain at home.

- The pain of pleurisy gets worse with a deep breath or cough. Call your doctor.

- If the pain throbs with each heartbeat, the covering of the heart may be inflamed (pericarditis). Call your doctor.

- Pain from an ulcer is worse on an empty stomach and gets better with food. Call your doctor.

- Pain from the gallbladder is often more intense after a meal. Call your doctor.

HOME TREATMENT

Treat pain in the chest wall with a pain reliever (p. 149) or topical treatments (e.g., Ben-Gay, Vicks Vaporub). Rest and heat will also help. See the doctor if chest pain lasts for more than five days.

WHAT TO EXPECT

The doctor will take the history and do a physical examination. Most likely, the doctor will run an electrocardiogram (EKG) and blood tests. The doctor may do additional tests if the cause of chest pain remains unknown. The person with chest pain may need to stay in the hospital. The doctor may prescribe pain medication.

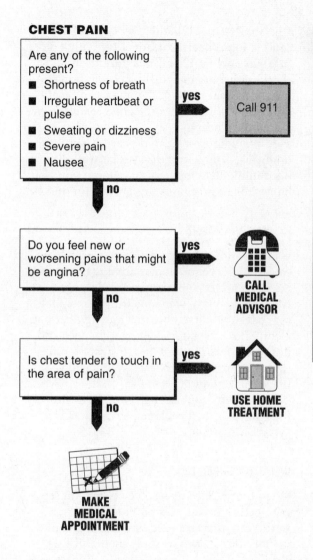

CHEST PAIN

Are any of the following present?
- Shortness of breath
- Irregular heartbeat or pulse
- Sweating or dizziness
- Severe pain
- Nausea

yes → Call 911

no ↓

Do you feel new or worsening pains that might be angina?

yes → **CALL MEDICAL ADVISOR**

no ↓

Is chest tender to touch in the area of pain?

yes → **USE HOME TREATMENT**

no ↓

MAKE MEDICAL APPOINTMENT

HEART ATTACK

The chest pain of a heart attack is usually intense, though it can be mild. Sometimes the sensation is more like pressure or squeezing on the chest. Usually the pain or discomfort is centered beneath the breastbone. The pain may radiate to the jaw or down the inner part of either arm.

A person having a heart attack may experience nausea, sweating, dizziness, or shortness of breath. Call 911 immediately if you suspect a heart attack.

Chest pain that occurs with exertion and goes away with rest isn't an actual heart attack. Doctors call this angina pectoris, or angina. The risk of a heart attack is highest when you feel new or worse angina pain. Call your doctor immediately if you have new angina pains.

SHORTNESS OF BREATH AND PALPITATIONS

Being winded or breathless after strenuous physical activity is normal. This isn't what doctors mean by "shortness of breath." Shortness of breath is a problem if you:

- Get winded after only slight exertion or at rest
- Wake up in the night out of breath
- Sleep propped up on several pillows to breathe easily

These are serious symptoms that require prompt medical attention.

Wheezing (p. 38) is noisy breathing, with difficulty exhaling. Wheezing may suggest asthma or another long-lasting condition.

The hyperventilation syndrome (p. 109) is a common cause of shortness of breath. The person has the sensation of shortness of breath but is actually overbreathing. He or she may also feel tingling in the fingers and toes and around the lips.

Nearly everybody has heart palpitations sometimes—a heartbeat that seems to suddenly start pounding, rapidly flutter, or skip a beat. These variations may result from exercise, intense emotions, or stress, or there may be no identifiable cause.

An occasional extra heartbeat is very common, felt as a flip-flop or thump in the chest. Most of the time this is completely harmless. Call the doctor if you feel more than five extra beats in a minute, or if they come in runs of three or more. Otherwise, mention this problem during your next medical appointment.

Anxiety (p. 112) and fever (p. 100) can cause a rapid heartbeat. An adult with a pulse that stays above 120 beats a minute should check with a doctor. Healthy children may have a normal pulse in that range and feel fine, but call the doctor if a child *complains* of a pounding heart.

Palpitations or a rapid heartbeat are seldom a sign of serious disease. However, you need immediate medical attention if you also have shortness of breath or chest pain (p. 84).

HOME TREATMENT

Usually, stress or some other minor problem causes hyperventilation and palpitations. It is important that you relax and rest.

If you believe someone is hyperventilating, have the person breathe into a paper bag. Gently hold the paper bag over the face and nose for a few minutes and, if hyperventilation is the problem, the symptoms will usually go away.

Talk with your doctor if you're unsure of the nature of the problem. See the doctor if symptoms persist.

WHAT TO EXPECT

Often the symptoms resolve before you see the doctor, so your description is very important. If your heart was racing, tell the doctor your pulse rate and whether it was regular.

The doctor will take a history and do a medical exam, paying particular attention to the heart, lungs, and breathing. He or she may request blood tests, chest X-rays, or an electrocardiogram (EKG).

The doctor may prescribe medication. Depending on the nature of the illness, you may stay in the hospital for observation or treatment.

SHORTNESS OF BREATH AND PALPITATIONS

Do you see any of these signs?
- Shortness of breath at rest
- Shortness of breath or chest pain with palpitations
- Wheezing

yes →

SEEK MEDICAL CARE NOW

no ↓

Is there shortness of breath with tingling in fingers, toes, or around mouth?

yes →

See: Hyperventilation (p. 109)

no ↓

Is either of the following present?
- Extra beats coming more than 4 per minute or in runs of 3 or more
- Pulse rate more than 120 beats per minute

yes →

SEEK MEDICAL CARE TODAY

no ↓

USE HOME TREATMENT

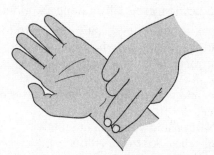

Wrist pulse. This drawing shows the technique for taking a pulse from the inside of the wrist. (*Caution:* Do not use your thumb, which has its own pulse.)

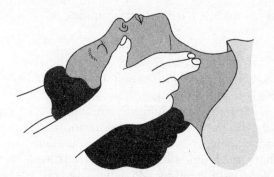

Neck pulse. This drawing shows the technique for taking a pulse from either side of the neck. (*Caution:* Do not take pulse from both sides of the neck at once.)

NAUSEA AND VOMITING

Nausea and vomiting have many causes. People often blame these stomach problems on food poisoning, though this is one of the less common causes. More likely are:

- Medication, especially among the elderly
- Viral infections, especially among children and young adults (who usually have diarrhea at the same time)

Ulcers and cancers are occasional causes of nausea.

Nausea and vomiting are rarely emergencies. See the doctor if:

- You are vomiting dark "coffee ground" material or bright red blood
- You have severe abdominal pain
- Nausea and vomiting follow a head injury
- You also have headache and a stiff neck
- A child with nausea and vomiting is lethargic or irritable

Call the doctor if you're pregnant, have diabetes, or take medication that might cause nausea and vomiting.

Severe and prolonged vomiting can lead to dehydration. How fast dehydration can develop depends on the person's size and how much fluid he or she loses. Diarrhea along with vomiting will dehydrate you quicker than either alone. See page 91 for more information on how to recognize and respond to this problem.

HOME TREATMENT

The goal of home treatment is to prevent dehydration. The person with nausea and vomiting should drink as much fluid as possible without upsetting the stomach any further.

Sip clear fluids such as water or ginger ale. Suck on ice chips if nothing else will stay down. Drink small amounts at a time, and avoid solid foods.

Try soups, bouillon, gelatin, and apple-sauce as you improve. Popsicles or iced fruit bars often work well with children. Milk products can sometimes make nausea and vomiting worse. Slowly work up to a normal diet.

Call the doctor if vomiting lasts for more than 72 hours, or if the person becomes dehydrated. Call the doctor if nausea lasts for four weeks. If a medication may be causing nausea or vomiting, ask your doctor whether you should keep taking it.

WHAT TO EXPECT

The doctor will take a history and physical examination, in particular assessing the person's hydration and looking for causes of nausea and vomiting. He or she may request blood tests, a urinalysis, and X-ray studies of the digestive tract to help diagnose the problem.

The doctor may start intravenous (IV) fluids if dehydration is severe. The person may need to stay in the hospital. The doctor may also prescribe medication to treat vomiting.

NAUSEA AND VOMITING

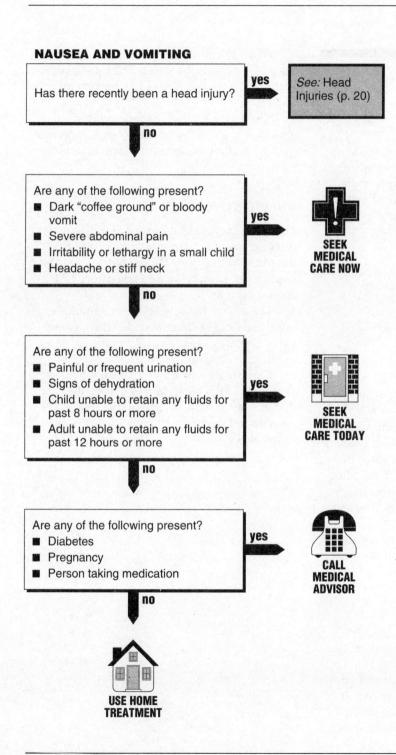

Has there recently been a head injury? **yes** → *See:* Head Injuries (p. 20)

no ↓

Are any of the following present?
- Dark "coffee ground" or bloody vomit
- Severe abdominal pain
- Irritability or lethargy in a small child
- Headache or stiff neck

yes → **SEEK MEDICAL CARE NOW**

no ↓

Are any of the following present?
- Painful or frequent urination
- Signs of dehydration
- Child unable to retain any fluids for past 8 hours or more
- Adult unable to retain any fluids for past 12 hours or more

yes → **SEEK MEDICAL CARE TODAY**

no ↓

Are any of the following present?
- Diabetes
- Pregnancy
- Person taking medication

yes → **CALL MEDICAL ADVISOR**

no ↓

USE HOME TREATMENT

DIARRHEA

Viruses, bacteria, and food poisoning are common causes of diarrhea. Several digestive disorders also cause chronic diarrhea, or diarrhea that alternates with constipation.

Many medications cause diarrhea, including:

- Nonsteroidal anti-inflammatory drugs (NSAIDs), especially meclofenamate (Meclomen)
- Antibiotics
- Gold compounds
- Blood pressure drugs
- Digitalis
- Anticancer drugs

Usually diarrhea is mild and improves within a few days of home treatment. Black or bloody diarrhea suggests bleeding from the digestive tract that needs a doctor's attention. However, medicines containing bismuth subsalicylate (e.g., Pepto-Bismol) or iron can also turn the stool black.

Cramping and gaslike pains are common with diarrhea. See the doctor if you have severe abdominal pain.

HOME TREATMENT

The goal of home treatment is to take in as much fluid as possible without upsetting the intestinal tract any further. Pedialyte is essential for infants. Older children and adults should sip clear fluids. Tap water is best. If nothing will stay down, try sucking on ice chips. Children should avoid juices or soda.

When the situation has improved, introduce bland foods: bananas, rice, applesauce, and toast. Avoid milk and fats for several days.

You may get relief from nonprescription remedies such as Pepto-Bismol or Kaopectate (p. 159). Call your doctor if diarrhea lasts for more than 96 hours.

WHAT TO EXPECT

The doctor will take a history and do a physical exam to assess hydration and find the cause of diarrhea. He or she may request blood tests, urinalysis, and laboratory tests on a stool sample.

The doctor may prescribe an antibiotic, but these drugs often make diarrhea worse. He or she may also prescribe a narcotic-like medication to treat diarrhea.

Chronic diarrhea may require more evaluation. If dehydration is severe, the doctor may give intravenous (IV) fluids. The dehydrated person may have to stay in the hospital.

DIARRHEA

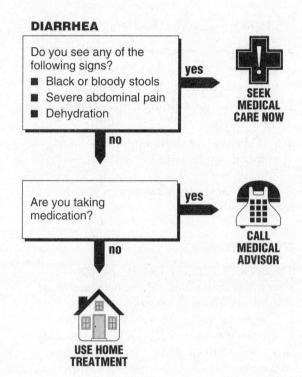

Do you see any of the following signs?
- Black or bloody stools
- Severe abdominal pain
- Dehydration

yes → SEEK MEDICAL CARE NOW

no

Are you taking medication?

yes → CALL MEDICAL ADVISOR

no

USE HOME TREATMENT

DEHYDRATION

Severe and prolonged diarrhea can lead to dehydration. Fever and vomiting increase fluid loss and raise the risk of dehydration. People with the lowest tolerance for dehydration are infants, the elderly, and those with health problems. Signs of dehydration are:

- Marked thirst
- Scanty urination or dark yellow urine
- Dry mouth
- Eyes that appear sunken
- Skin that has lost its normal elasticity. Normally skin springs back if you pinch it; when a person is dehydrated the skin may remain tented up after pinching.

Heartburn

Heartburn is the irritation of the esophagus (passage from mouth to stomach) by gastric juices. These juices, produced in the stomach, aid in digestion and are strong acids.

The stomach lining normally protects against gastric acid. (Bacterial infection causes many of the painful ulcers in the stomach or small intestine.)

Unlike the stomach, however, the esophagus is not protected against acid. Backflow of acid from the stomach irritates the lining of the esophagus. We call this gastroesophageal reflux (GER). Usually the discomfort is worse when you lie down.

Smoking, caffeine, aspirin, stress, and other factors can make the digestive tract more vulnerable to heartburn.

Call the doctor if you vomit dark "coffee ground" material or bright red blood, or if you have black, tarry stools. However, iron supplements and bismuth subsalicylate (Pepto-Bismol) can also cause black stools.

HOME TREATMENT

Avoid substances that make heartburn worse, such as coffee, tea, alcohol, aspirin, ibuprofen, and naproxen. Think about the effects of smoking and stress.

You may get relief from an antacid such as Maalox, Mylanta, Tums, or Gelusil (p. 158). You can substitute nonfat milk for antacid. You can also try a nonprescription acid blocker such as Tagamet or Pepcid AC (p. 158). Baking soda can give quick relief but you shouldn't use it repeatedly.

Here are some tips for reducing reflux:

- Avoid lying down or reclining after eating.
- Elevate the head of the bed with blocks four to six inches (10 to 15 cm).
- Don't wear tight-fitting clothes (girdles, tight jeans).
- Avoid eating or drinking for two hours before going to bed.

Call your doctor if heartburn lasts for more than three days.

WHAT TO EXPECT

The doctor will take a history and do a physical exam to find out the nature of your discomfort. He or she may request X-rays of the digestive tract, which could include swallowing barium. Called a GI (gastrointestinal) series, this painless procedure helps diagnose ulcers, hernia, reflux, and other digestive disorders.

Unless you are bleeding in the digestive tract, treatment is conservative. If you have a gastric acid problem, the doctor will likely suggest a therapy similar to the home treatment we describe. He or she may prescribe other medication to reduce stomach acid or reflux. The doctor may prescribe an oral antibiotic to treat ulcers.

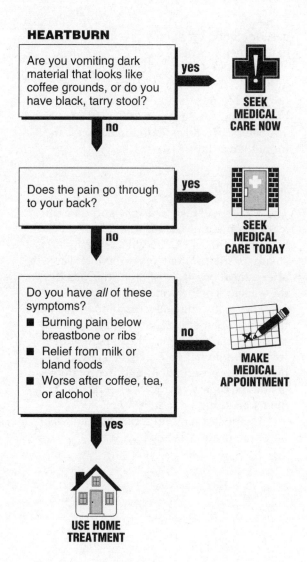

HEARTBURN

Are you vomiting dark material that looks like coffee grounds, or do you have black, tarry stool?

→ **yes** → **SEEK MEDICAL CARE NOW**

↓ **no**

Does the pain go through to your back?

→ **yes** → **SEEK MEDICAL CARE TODAY**

↓ **no**

Do you have *all* of these symptoms?
- Burning pain below breastbone or ribs
- Relief from milk or bland foods
- Worse after coffee, tea, or alcohol

→ **no** → **MAKE MEDICAL APPOINTMENT**

↓ **yes**

USE HOME TREATMENT

ABDOMINAL PAIN

Abdominal pain can signal a serious condition, but most of the time the problem is minor. The organs of the abdomen can cause a range of different pains and sensations. The pain may be intermittent (like "gas") or more steady.

Ulcers tend to cause burning pain in the upper abdomen that gets better after a meal or a dose of antacid. A bacterium called helicobacter pylori causes many stomach ulcers. Talk to your doctor if your pain lasts for a couple of weeks.

If you have pain that recurs with the menstrual cycle, talk to your doctor. Abdominal pain during pregnancy is potentially serious and requires medical attention. A woman can have the pain from an ectopic pregnancy—a fertilized egg in the fallopian tube rather than in the uterus—before she is aware she is pregnant.

Call the doctor if you:

- Have severe abdominal pain
- Have bleeding from the bowel
- Had a recent abdominal injury
- Are or may be pregnant

HOME TREATMENT

Persistent abdominal pain requires medical attention. Use home treatment for mild pains that resolve within 24 hours or are due to stomach flu, heartburn, or other minor problems.

Sip water or other clear fluids, but avoid solid foods. A bowel movement, passage of gas, or a good belch may give relief. A warm bath sometimes helps.

You can take an antacid for heartburn, indigestion, or suspected stomach ulcer (p. 158). If antacids don't work, try an acid blocker, such as Tagamet or Pepcid AC.

See the doctor if abdominal pain lasts more than a day or two.

WHAT TO EXPECT

The doctor will take a history and do a physical examination. The location of the pain will be significant, as will be whether the pain is steady or intermittent, and whether it lessens after a meal or a dose of antacid. Consider these factors beforehand.

The doctor may also run blood tests and a urinalysis. Sometimes X-ray studies of the abdomen may be done. The person with severe abdominal pain may be kept in the hospital for observation. Endoscopy (looking inside the digestive tract with a flexible tube) may sometimes be required.

The doctor may prescribe antibiotics or other medication as needed.

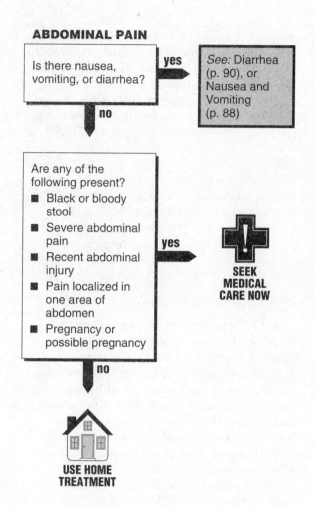

ABDOMINAL PAIN

Is there nausea, vomiting, or diarrhea? — **yes** → *See:* Diarrhea (p. 90), or Nausea and Vomiting (p. 88)

no ↓

Are any of the following present?

- Black or bloody stool
- Severe abdominal pain
- Recent abdominal injury
- Pain localized in one area of abdomen
- Pregnancy or possible pregnancy

yes → **SEEK MEDICAL CARE NOW**

no ↓

USE HOME TREATMENT

APPENDICITIS

An inflamed appendix is a serious problem, but most pains in the abdomen have other causes. The most reliable signal of appendicitis is the *order* in which symptoms develop:

1. Pain—usually around the belly button or just below the breastbone at first
2. Loss of appetite, nausea, or vomiting
3. Tenderness in the right lower abdomen
4. Fever of 100°F to 102°F (38°C to 39°C)

Appendicitis is unlikely if fever or vomiting comes before the initial pain.

CONSTIPATION AND RECTAL PAIN

Many people worry too much about bowel habits—the frequency, consistency, and color of stool. Rectal problems are usually minor, though they may be uncomfortable and interfere with your quality of life.

There is no "normal" for bowel movements. Having bowel movements three times a day—or once every three days—can be normal for you. Stool may change in color, texture, consistency, or bulk. Some people are regular, some are not. You shouldn't worry unless there is a major change from what is normal for you. Even then, it is rare for a change in bowel habits to signal a serious problem.

Make an appointment with the doctor if you're losing weight or have thin, pencil-like stools. Call the doctor if you have pain or swelling of the abdomen, or if symptoms last more than a week.

Hemorrhoids

Hemorrhoids (piles) are the most common rectal problem. A hemorrhoid is an enlargement of the veins around the anus, similar to a varicose vein. These veins tend to enlarge with age, particularly among those who sit a lot. Straining at bowel movements can irritate the veins, resulting in pain and tenderness. The pain and inflammation usually go away within a few days or weeks. After healing, a small flap or tag of tissue often remains.

You may be worried by seeing blood with your stool. If the bleeding is bright red and relatively light, it probably is coming from hemorrhoids or the lower intestine. This isn't medically significant unless it persists for several weeks. If the blood is dark, or turns the stool burgundy or black, the bleeding has happened higher in the digestive tract. You should take this signal seriously. Iron supplements and bismuth subsalicylate (Pepto-Bismol) can also turn the stool black.

Pinworms

The pinworm is a parasite that can infect the rectum and cause rectal pain and itching. This is most common in children. Pinworms occasionally infect the vagina. Your doctor can prescribe medication to treat pinworms.

HOME TREATMENT

Dietary fiber is important to good bowel health. Fiber draws water into the digestive tract, adding bulk and softening the stool. A high-fiber diet not only prevents constipation but also may reduce your risk of hemorrhoids, diverticulosis, intestinal polyps, and colon cancer. Fiber is often absent from heavily processed foods. For fiber, your diet should contain fresh fruits and vegetables, bran, and whole-grain bread.

If you must use laxatives, we prefer a bulk laxative such as Metamucil (p. 159). An enema (e.g., Fleet's) may help occasional, severe constipation. Talk to your doctor if you need an enema more than once in a while.

For hemorrhoids, keep the area clean. Wash regularly in the shower, or use a washcloth. Avoid vigorous wiping with toilet paper. Zinc oxide paste or powder (p. 157) will help protect hemorrhoids from further irritation. Hemorrhoid remedies are also available over the counter. We advise against using products containing an anesthetic, which can irritate the area and delay healing. A soothing suppository may help internal

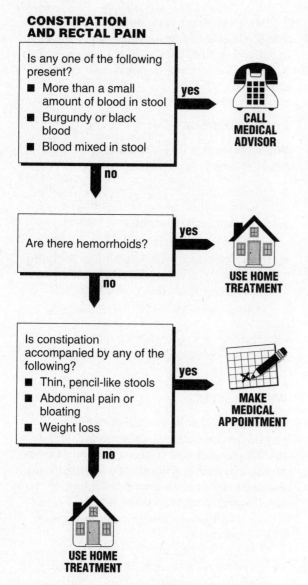

CONSTIPATION AND RECTAL PAIN

Is any one of the following present?
- More than a small amount of blood in stool
- Burgundy or black blood
- Blood mixed in stool

yes → **CALL MEDICAL ADVISOR**

no ↓

Are there hemorrhoids?

yes → **USE HOME TREATMENT**

no ↓

Is constipation accompanied by any of the following?
- Thin, pencil-like stools
- Abdominal pain or bloating
- Weight loss

yes → **MAKE MEDICAL APPOINTMENT**

no ↓

USE HOME TREATMENT

hemorrhoids. See the doctor if you aren't completely relieved in a week. Even if the problem goes away, mention it during your next office visit.

WHAT TO EXPECT

The doctor will take the history and do a physical examination. If you have had a major change in bowel habits, the doctor may do a rectal examination or examine the colon with a flexible tube (sigmoidoscope). He or she may order X-rays of the lower bowel, which may require a barium enema.

If a clot has formed in a hemorrhoid, the doctor may lance the vein and remove the clot. Hemorrhoids seldom need surgery, which is reserved for persistent problems.

DIFFICULT URINATION

The signs of urinary bladder inflammation are:

- Painful or burning urination
- Frequent, urgent urination
- Blood in the urine

Bacterial infection most often causes bladder inflammation. Symptoms may also be caused by a virus or by drinking a lot of caffeinated beverages (some—but not all—coffee, tea, and soft drinks).

Bladder infection is far more common in women than it is in men. The urethra is much shorter in females, giving germs a smaller distance to travel to the bladder. Wiping from front to back after defecating helps prevent bladder infections. Sexual activity can cause bladder infection among females. Bladder infections are common during pregnancy—and more difficult for the doctor to treat.

In men, symptoms similar to bladder infection can be caused by infection of the prostate (prostatitis), an enlarged prostate (benign prostatic hypertrophy, or BPH), and prostate cancer. These symptoms include difficulty in starting urination, dribbling, or decreased force of the urinary stream. Most elderly men have these symptoms to some degree. Distinguishing bladder infection from prostate disorders can be difficult. See the doctor if home treatment doesn't quickly relieve the symptoms.

Most bacterial bladder infections respond to home treatment. Still, many doctors give antibiotics to patients, particularly women with repeated bladder infections.

Microbes that infect the bladder can pass into the kidney. Symptoms of kidney infection include vomiting, back pain, and severe chills. Kidney infection requires immediate medical attention.

HOME TREATMENT

When you notice the symptoms of bacterial infection, start home treatment:

- Drink as much as you can—up to a gallon or more of fluid in the first 24 hours. This will make copious urine and literally wash the bacteria out of your body.
- Drink fruit juices. This puts more acid into the urine, which may help bring relief. Cranberry juice is the most effective because it contains a natural antibiotic.

Call the doctor if you aren't a lot better within 24 hours and completely well within 48 hours.

WHAT TO EXPECT

The doctor will take your history and do a physical examination. Lab personnel will do a urinalysis and urine culture (sometimes these tests are available without you having to see the doctor). The doctor will do a more detailed workup and run more tests if you have a history of kidney disease or symptoms of kidney infection.

Men with symptoms of prostate disease can expect a rectal exam. The doctor may then suggest drug therapy, "watchful waiting," or one of several surgical options to treat symptoms of prostate disease.

For women, the doctor may do a pelvic exam and additional tests if there is a vaginal discharge (p. 120).

If urine tests show bacterial infection, the doctor will prescribe an antibiotic.

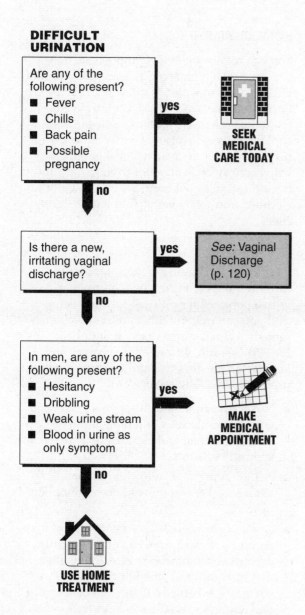

DIFFICULT URINATION

Are any of the following present?
- Fever
- Chills
- Back pain
- Possible pregnancy

yes → **SEEK MEDICAL CARE TODAY**

no ↓

Is there a new, irritating vaginal discharge?

yes → *See:* Vaginal Discharge (p. 120)

no ↓

In men, are any of the following present?
- Hesitancy
- Dribbling
- Weak urine stream
- Blood in urine as only symptom

yes → **MAKE MEDICAL APPOINTMENT**

no ↓

USE HOME TREATMENT

FEVER

A high temperature is not always a sign of illness. Normal body temperature varies from person to person, and is usually lower in the morning. Physical activity, excitement, anxiety, food, and heavy clothing can all raise body temperature. Hormones can cause a monthly change in body temperature in fertile women. Children usually have a higher temperature than adults, and their temperatures go up and down more during the day.

The point at which an elevated temperature becomes a fever is not well-defined. To make it easy, we say that a fever is a temperature over 100°F (38°C) taken with an oral thermometer. A temperature that remains around 99 to 100°F (38°C) for a week or more also deserves attention.

Causes

The most common causes of fever are viral and bacterial infections, such as colds, sore throats, earaches, diarrhea, urinary infections, roseola, chicken pox, mumps, and measles. Pneumonia, appendicitis, and meningitis are also occasional causes.

A fever can cause the brain's temperature center to register cold, triggering the body's systems to produce more heat, such as by shivering. The person with fever may look pale, as blood is shunted away from the skin. He or she may have goose bumps. Children will sometimes curl up in a ball to conserve heat. Don't bundle up the person with chills in blankets. This will only cause the fever to go higher.

HOME TREATMENT

You can reduce the body temperature of a person with a high fever by sponging the skin with lukewarm water. (Cool water may be uncomfortable. Do not use alcohol because the fumes can be dangerous.) You can also cool the person in a tub of water about 70°F (21°C). Wetting the hair will feel good and help carry away heat. After drying, have the person rest in a cool room wearing little or no clothing. You can cover a child with a light sheet.

Medication

You don't need to do anything for a mild fever. If the fever is high enough to interfere with a person's sleep, work, or other activities, you can treat it with an over-the-counter remedy. We recommend acetaminophen (p. 149). Aspirin, ibuprofen, naproxen, and ketoprofen are also safe and effective when used properly. Remember:

- Never give oral medication to a person who is unconscious or having a seizure. Acetaminophen and aspirin are available in suppository form.

- Avoid giving aspirin to children or teenagers. We recommend acetaminophen instead.

- Use all drugs carefully, whether or not they require a prescription. Never take a drug prescribed to somebody else. Remember that medications come in different strengths. Mixing up drugs can be dangerous, especially for children.

Starve a Fever?

You may have heard the old saying that begins, "Starve a fever . . . ." Unfortunately, it's not a helpful old saying. There are many

SEIZURES

An extremely high fever can cause a seizure or convulsion. Such seizures are relatively common in normal, healthy children, especially those between six months and four years of age. Although a seizure may appear dramatic, there is little danger to the child. Usually a fever-related seizure lasts a few minutes and causes no lasting effects. (Sometimes there is brief weakness or even paralysis in an arm or leg.) Less than half of all children who have one such seizure ever have another. Repeated seizures, or a seizure that lasts more than 30 minutes, may suggest more serious medical conditions.

If a child with a fever has seizures, do the following:

- Protect his or her head from hitting the floor or hard objects. Place the child on a bed.

- Keep the child's airway open, and do rescue breathing as needed.

- Do not force an object or your fingers into a person's mouth. This is likely to result in injury. It's not possible for the child to "swallow the tongue," and serious tongue bites are rare.

- Start to lower the child's fever with sponging or suppositories (p. 151). Never give a person having seizures anything by mouth, such as liquids or medication.

- **Get immediate medical attention.** Call 911 if necessary.

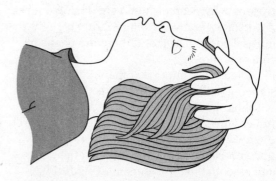

Open airway. If a child is having a febrile seizure, pull the head back slightly. Do not force anything into the mouth.

reasons why people should eat during a fever. A person whose body temperature is high burns calories faster, and therefore needs to consume more.

Even more important than food for someone with a fever are fluids. Never withhold liquids from a feverish person (unless he or she is in the middle of a seizure). Even if the fever makes the person so uncomfortable that he or she won't eat, it is still essential that the person drink fluids.

Call the doctor if a fever lasts for more than 48 hours, or if it stays above 103°F (39.5°C) after an hour of home treatment.

WHAT TO EXPECT

The medical professional will take a history and do a physical examination to assess fever and other symptoms. If a person appears very sick, doctors may run blood and urine tests. In rare cases, a doctor may order a chest X-ray. If the person has had a seizure for the first time, a doctor may order a spinal tap to check for meningitis. If you have a bacterial infection, a doctor or nurse-practitioner may prescribe an antibiotic.

Often the medical professional will suggest sponging or over-the-counter medication, as we describe above. If you have no infection or other symptoms, the doctor may advise "watchful waiting."

HEAT STROKE

Exposure to a warm and humid environment, especially while not drinking enough fluids, can cause heat exhaustion. Symptoms include weakness, headache, dizziness, thirst, nausea, and vomiting. The person's temperature may be elevated, but not above 101°F (38°C). The skin of a person with heat exhaustion is sweaty because the body is trying to cool off. Move the person into a cool place and have him or her drink lots of water.

Heat stroke, also called sun stroke, is an **emergency.** It arises when the body is no longer able to cool off. A person with heat stroke has dry skin. Body temperature rises quickly when sweating stops, even topping 105°F (40.5°C). A person suffering heat stroke no longer complains of heat or thirst. He or she may be confused or delirious, lose consciousness, or have seizures.

The person with heat stroke needs immediate medical care. You must rapidly cool the person's body by ice baths, ice packs, wet sheets, or any other means possible. Brain damage and other injuries may result if the victim's temperature doesn't go down. Treatment in the emergency room can be very effective.

FEVER

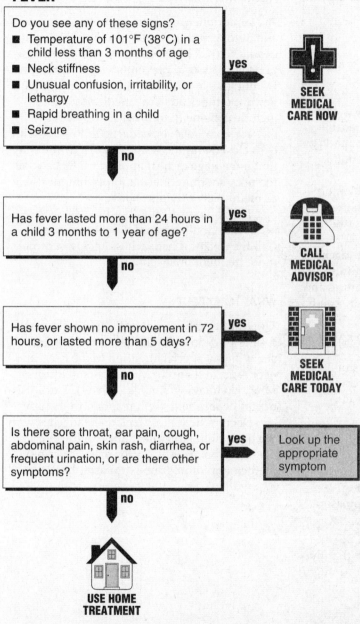

Do you see any of these signs?
- Temperature of 101°F (38°C) in a child less than 3 months of age
- Neck stiffness
- Unusual confusion, irritability, or lethargy
- Rapid breathing in a child
- Seizure

yes → **SEEK MEDICAL CARE NOW**

no

Has fever lasted more than 24 hours in a child 3 months to 1 year of age?

yes → **CALL MEDICAL ADVISOR**

no

Has fever shown no improvement in 72 hours, or lasted more than 5 days?

yes → **SEEK MEDICAL CARE TODAY**

no

Is there sore throat, ear pain, cough, abdominal pain, skin rash, diarrhea, or frequent urination, or are there other symptoms?

yes → Look up the appropriate symptom

no

USE HOME TREATMENT

HEADACHE

Headache is the single most common complaint of modern times. Usually tension and muscle spasms in the neck, scalp, and jaw cause headaches. They are annoying but invariably get better with time.

If your headaches are worse in the morning, consider having your blood pressure measured. High blood pressure can cause headaches.

Migraines are a type of severe headache causing pain on one side of the head only. A migraine often causes nausea or vomiting and may be preceded by flashes of light or seeing "stars."

Some people prone to headaches worry that they have a brain tumor. Unless you have some other dramatic signs—paralysis or a personality change—the chance that an occasional headache is a brain tumor is exceedingly remote.

When accompanied by other symptoms, a headache might be the sign of an **emergency:**

- After a head injury, a headache accompanied by vomiting or difficulty seeing suggests a dangerous increase in pressure inside the skull.

- A headache, fever, and the inability to touch the chin to the chest suggest that the covering of the brain and spinal cord might be inflamed (meningitis).

- Headaches that are accompanied by difficulty in using the arms or legs, or with slurring of speech, require immediate medical attention.

HOME TREATMENT

Acetaminophen, aspirin, ibuprofen, naproxen, and ketoprofen are quite effective in relieving headache (p. 149). You can take these medications with food to prevent stomach irritation. Do not give aspirin to children or teenagers. For migraine headaches, medications that include caffeine (Excedrin) are often best.

You may relieve headache by resting with eyes closed and the head supported. You may find a massage or heat applied to the back of the neck soothing. Relaxation techniques such as meditation may also work.

Talk to your doctor about persistent headaches that don't respond to home treatment. Call the doctor if headaches quickly become more frequent or severe.

WHAT TO EXPECT

The health professional will ask for a medical history and do a physical examination. He or she will pay special attention to the head and neck, and to neurological function. Doctors rarely do imaging studies such as CT or MRI unless headache doesn't respond to therapy.

Doctors treat most tension headaches with the basic home treatment approach we describe above. Your doctor may prescribe medication for migraine or cluster headache.

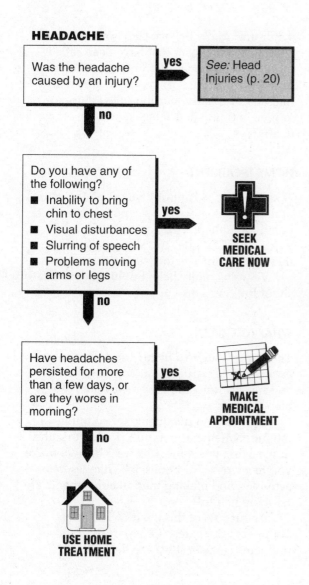

HEADACHE

Was the headache caused by an injury? — **yes** → *See:* Head Injuries (p. 20)

no

Do you have any of the following?
- Inability to bring chin to chest
- Visual disturbances
- Slurring of speech
- Problems moving arms or legs

yes → **SEEK MEDICAL CARE NOW**

no

Have headaches persisted for more than a few days, or are they worse in morning? — **yes** → **MAKE MEDICAL APPOINTMENT**

no

USE HOME TREATMENT

COMPUTER SYMPTOMS

Headache is just one of the symptoms that people who use computers for many hours at a time can develop. Staring at a computer screen for a long time can cause eye strain, irritation, blurred vision, and headaches. These problems are temporary. To reduce the risk of eye strain:

- Blink often, and use eye drops to keep your eyes wet. Rest your eyes with frequent glances away from the screen.

- Avoid glare from the screen by using indirect lighting, repositioning the screen, or using an antiglare filter.

- Make sure your monitor produces sharp, crisp images. Fuzzy screen images increase eye strain.

- Get special glasses for your computer work if necessary. If you wear bifocals, you may be tilting your head at an uncomfortable angle to see through the lower portion of your glasses.

Other computer users experience arm or back pains, which can also be avoided.

- Proper typing position is with your elbows at a 90° angle, your forearms parallel to the floor. Keep your wrists in a neutral position, and your feet flat on the floor.

- Use a wrist rest for support. Consider using a different keyboard.

- Though you may feel pressure to type without interruption, take brief rests.

WEAKNESS AND FATIGUE

Weakness is a lack of *strength*, while fatigue is a lack of *energy*. Weakness is the more serious condition, especially when it is confined to one area of the body. That is often due to a muscular or nervous system problem, such as a stroke.

Fatigue is tiredness, lethargy, or a lack of energy. About one in every four adults seen in a doctor's office complain of chronic fatigue. The symptom may be associated with a range of conditions and illness, including viral infection, anxiety, or tension. Here are some of the causes people ask about most often:

- Low blood sugar (hypoglycemia) makes a few people feel shaky several hours after a meal, but is rarely the cause of feeling tired throughout the day.

- Iron deficiency (anemia) causes only a small number of fatigue cases.

- Thyroid problems also are a rare cause.

- Sleep apnea produces fatigue in people who snore or find themselves waking up many times in the night (p. 116).

- Fibromyalgia is a rare cause (p. 66).

- Depression often makes people feel tired but is less likely to cause fatigue than to result from fatigue that has been caused by other factors (p. 114).

Of all the people who complain of chronic fatigue, perhaps only one in a thousand meets the criteria for what doctors have come to recognize as chronic fatigue syndrome (CFS). Doctors are still debating the cause of this syndrome. Many believe CFS is actually a collection of diseases that have been called different things over the centuries. There is now a standard list of criteria doctors use to diagnose the rare condition called chronic fatigue immune-deficiency syndrome (CFIDS).

HOME TREATMENT

Take the time to carefully reflect on the causes of fatigue. Usually, poor sleeping habits, boredom, unhappiness, or just plain hard work causes fatigue. You should consider these possibilities before seeing the doctor.

Vitamins rarely help, but in moderation shouldn't hurt you.

WHAT TO EXPECT

The doctor will do a history and physical exam, paying particular attention to nerve and muscle function. He or she may request blood tests.

There are no treatments for common fatigue. Caffeine or pep pills don't work; the downswing when the pills wear off will make you feel worse. Vacations, job changes, new activities, and making marital adjustments are far more helpful.

About 80% of those with CFS suffer depression or anxiety. Often, treating those problems is the best way to deal with CFS.

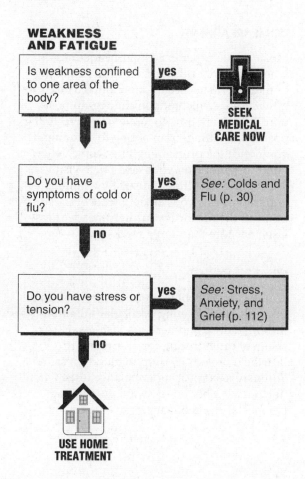

**WEAKNESS
AND FATIGUE**

Is weakness confined to one area of the body?

yes → SEEK MEDICAL CARE NOW

no ↓

Do you have symptoms of cold or flu?

yes → *See:* Colds and Flu (p. 30)

no ↓

Do you have stress or tension?

yes → *See:* Stress, Anxiety, and Grief (p. 112)

no ↓

USE HOME TREATMENT

DIZZINESS AND FAINTING

Losing consciousness, with no control over your body and no memory of the event, is a serious problem. It should be investigated promptly by a doctor. If you can't rouse an unconscious person, that is an **emergency.**

A "blackout" in which you feel dizzy and need to sit or lie down but can still hear is not a full loss of consciousness. Such blackouts (or gray-outs) are often related to changes of posture or emotional experiences. Dizziness and feeling light-headed are similar problems, usually not serious, though you can fall and hurt yourself during an episode.

Vertigo is a disorder of the balance mechanism of the inner ear. You experience a loss of balance and, because the balance mechanism helps control eye movements, the room seems to spin or lurch crazily. Most vertigo has no definite cause. You should see a doctor with this symptom.

Light-headedness is a woozy feeling. It is the most common and least serious form of dizziness. It can have many causes:

- Colds and flu (p. 30)
- Anxiety
- Standing or sitting up quickly if you have low blood pressure; gravity momentarily halts blood flow to the brain, resulting in loss of vision and light-headedness
- Medications (call the prescribing doctor if you feel this side effect)
- Alcohol (see page 118 for advice on excess drinking)

HOME TREATMENT

Most people experience light-headedness when suddenly raising their head or getting to their feet. This occurs more often as we grow older. Avoid sudden changes in position. Take more time to move from a reclining position to sitting, from sitting to standing. If you notice the problem getting worse, tell your doctor during your next office visit.

Light-headedness caused by emotions will improve as your anxiety resolves.

Call the doctor if your light-headedness lasts for more than three weeks.

WHAT TO EXPECT

The doctor will obtain your history and do a physical exam, paying particular attention to the circulatory and nervous systems. He or she may order testing for an irregular heartbeat or sudden drop in blood pressure. You may need hearing or balance tests. Often doctors try a period of "watchful waiting" before starting more aggressive treatment.

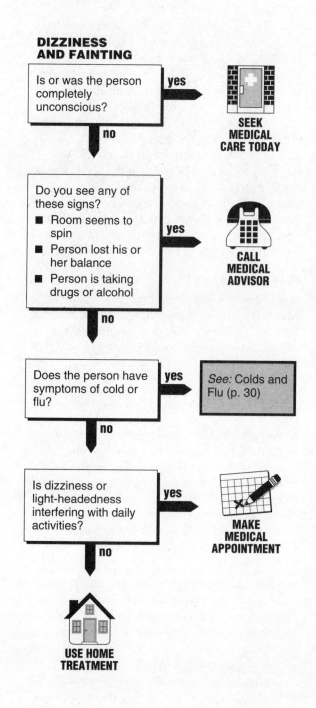

DIZZINESS AND FAINTING

Is or was the person completely unconscious?

yes → SEEK MEDICAL CARE TODAY

no ↓

Do you see any of these signs?
- Room seems to spin
- Person lost his or her balance
- Person is taking drugs or alcohol

yes → CALL MEDICAL ADVISOR

no ↓

Does the person have symptoms of cold or flu?

yes → *See:* Colds and Flu (p. 30)

no ↓

Is dizziness or light-headedness interfering with daily activities?

yes → MAKE MEDICAL APPOINTMENT

no ↓

USE HOME TREATMENT

HYPERVENTILATION

Some people feel dizzy during episodes of hyperventilation, or "panic attack." Hyperventilation is the most troubling symptom of anxiety. The person feels unable to get enough air into his or her lungs, and becomes concerned about breathing. The hyperventilating person may feel chest pain and tightness, dizziness, muscle spasm, and a tingling or numb sensation in the hands and feet. The person may think he or she is having a heart attack or a nervous breakdown. These feelings result not from a lack of oxygen but from a loss of carbon dioxide caused by overbreathing.

Typically hyperventilation affects nervous and tense people. Alcohol, severe pain, or stressful situations may trigger the syndrome. A panic-prone person will likely have repeated attacks.

If the person is hyperventilating, have him or her breathe into a paper bag. Hold a paper bag loosely over the nose and mouth for five to 15 minutes. This will raise carbon dioxide levels in the blood and stop the attack. The victim must try to calm down. Give your reassurance. When the victim recognizes that the problem is anxiety and not a medical disease, the panic attacks will stop.

HIGH BLOOD PRESSURE

High blood pressure (hypertension) is one of the most common and most treatable chronic health problems. It affects 30 to 40 million Americans—more than one in ten. High blood pressure is a silent disease, often causing no symptoms until it is too late. A catastrophic heart attack, stroke, or kidney disease is often the first sign of disease.

Two numbers make up the blood pressure reading. The upper number, or systolic, represents the maximum pressure in the arteries when the heart pumps. The lower number, or diastolic, is the pressure while the heart is at rest.

A typical blood pressure may be 120/80, but what is "normal" varies over a wide range. In general, the lower the blood pressure, the better. Blood pressure is considered high if the upper (systolic) pressure is above 140, or if the lower (diastolic) number is above 90. Low readings are usually seen in children and adults in excellent physical condition.

Don't panic over one blood pressure result. Several readings over several weeks are needed to be meaningful. At least a third of those whose first reading is high have a normal reading when blood pressure is later rechecked.

Monitoring Your Blood Pressure

Have your blood pressure checked at least once a year. Blood pressure measurement is painless, quick, and reliable. The doctor's office may not be the best place to have your pressure checked, however, because being nervous can raise your blood pressure. Free blood pressure checks are often available at health fairs, businesses, and health agencies. Many stores, such as drug stores, have blood pressure machines available for public use, and these are reasonably accurate.

Is it worth buying a home blood pressure cuff or measuring machine? Many reliable, affordable models are on the market. If you have high blood pressure you'll want to check yourself frequently so you can report any changes or difficulties to your doctor; a home blood pressure monitor may make sense for you. But unless you intend to use a monitor frequently, it may not be worth the cost.

If You Have High Blood Pressure

It is important to understand that you must manage high blood pressure yourself. You bear the responsibility for controlling your weight, maintaining a proper level of activity, not smoking, limiting the salt and fats in your diet, and taking your medicine properly. Expect only a few doctor appointments for this condition.

- **Keep in Shape** Make exercise, weight control, and a good diet part of your routine. Although a person in good shape can have high blood pressure, your risk is greater if you're overweight and out of shape. Reducing your weight is a reliable way of lowering your blood pressure. Exercise conditions your cardiovascular system.
- **Diet** Decreasing the salt, fat, and cholesterol in your diet and increasing the potassium and calcium help lower blood pressure and decrease the risk of heart disease.
- **Managing Drugs** If the doctor prescribes medication to control your blood pressure, understand how to manage the drugs. Ask the doctor about side effects and warning

signs. On a chart, note which drugs you take, along with all your blood pressure measurements. With this record you and your doctor can make the important decisions about managing your high blood pressure.

Drug therapy is effective but is expensive and has risks and side effects. Through good self-care and risk reduction, many people can control their blood pressure without the need for medication. Others can reduce the drug dosage required to control the blood pressure, saving money as well as lowering risks and side effects. Aim to reduce your drug intake—but don't change your therapy unless your doctor says so.

■ **Stick With It** Managing high blood pressure is a lifelong job. Don't stop your program because you feel good. Don't wait for signs and symptoms before you take preventive measures. If you take care of high blood pressure, it will probably never cause you a major problem. If you ignore it, you are needlessly endangering your life and well-being.

STRESS, ANXIETY, AND GRIEF

Stress isn't a disease, but a fact of life. Our reactions can vary tremendously, sometimes in ways that are not good.

Anxiety is a common reaction to powerful stress, such as money troubles. People who react to daily stress with anxiety probably need counseling, though they may not realize that. They may instead focus on the common symptoms of anxiety:

- Insomnia
- Nervousness
- Rapid heart rate
- Inability to concentrate
- "Lump in the throat," or even difficulty swallowing
- Hyperventilation (like "lump in the throat," most common in young adults, especially women—see page 109)

Grief is a normal reaction to loss, such as the death of a loved one or the end of a job. Working through grief is an important part of dealing with loss. While family and community resources can provide some support, the only therapy for grief is time.

A grieving person may turn to alcohol, tranquilizers, or other prescription medication. While drugs may give short-term relief, they don't solve problems. Alcohol and drugs are crutches that interfere with normal recovery. You must address the underlying issues.

HOME TREATMENT

Recognizing the signs of anxiety is the first step to finding and treating its cause. You may find it helpful to talk with friends, family, or a member of the clergy. Agencies in your community provide services and referrals. Occasionally the person may require long-term therapy with a counselor. No single type of therapy is better for all people. Your choice should depend on what works for you.

Too much caffeine can cause chronic anxiety. Cutting down on caffeine may help you relax. Caffeine is found in coffee, soft drinks, tea, chocolate, nonprescription stimulants (e.g., No Doz, Vivarin), and a variety of cold and headache remedies.

Relaxation techniques and a program of regular physical exercise can help reduce anxiety.

WHAT TO EXPECT

For hyperventilation syndrome, the doctor may have the person breathe into a paper bag to restore normal breathing. The doctor may also ask the person to lie down and voluntarily hyperventilate (50 deep breaths) to understand how the symptoms arise. He or she may prescribe a tranquilizer.

The doctor will get the medical history and do a physical exam. Health providers may take an electrocardiogram (EKG) and chest X-rays. The doctor will evaluate anxiety and determine whether you need a referral to a mental health professional.

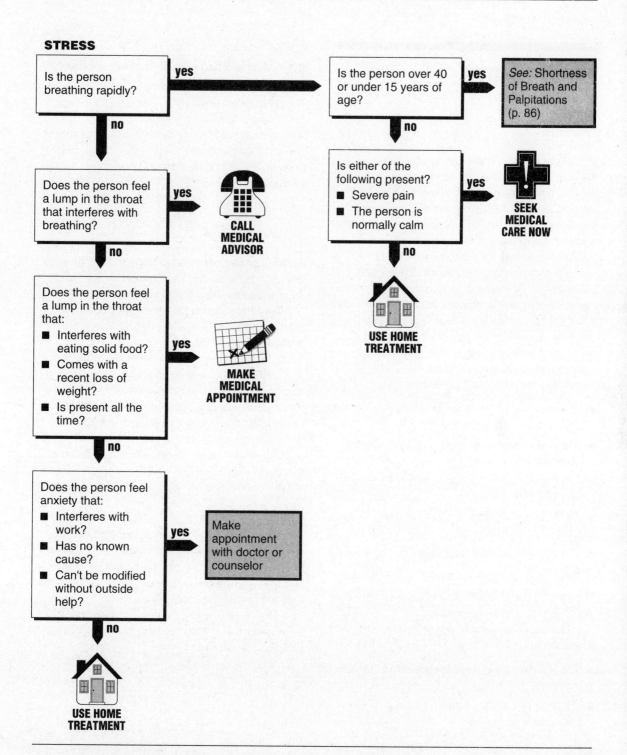

STRESS

Is the person breathing rapidly? — **yes** →

Is the person over 40 or under 15 years of age? — **yes** → *See:* Shortness of Breath and Palpitations (p. 86)

no ↓

no ↓

Does the person feel a lump in the throat that interferes with breathing? — **yes** → **CALL MEDICAL ADVISOR**

Is either of the following present?
■ Severe pain
■ The person is normally calm — **yes** → **SEEK MEDICAL CARE NOW**

no ↓

no ↓

USE HOME TREATMENT

Does the person feel a lump in the throat that:
■ Interferes with eating solid food?
■ Comes with a recent loss of weight?
■ Is present all the time? — **yes** → **MAKE MEDICAL APPOINTMENT**

no ↓

Does the person feel anxiety that:
■ Interferes with work?
■ Has no known cause?
■ Can't be modified without outside help? — **yes** → Make appointment with doctor or counselor

no ↓

USE HOME TREATMENT

DEPRESSION

Everybody gets the blues sometimes. Depression can range from a lack of energy to an overwhelming sense of hopelessness. It can seem like a general fatigue or a vague sense of ill health. You may feel poorly and not know why. The future holds no promise. You have a sense of loss.

Most depression is a normal response to an unhappy event. It is natural to be depressed by the death of a loved one, or after a big disappointment at work. However, if depression continues and starts to interfere with your work or family life, make an appointment to see your doctor.

Ask yourself these questions:

- Are you sad or blue for most of the day, for more days than not?
- Do you often cry even though you aren't sure why?
- Do you think that unhappiness is the rule in your life?
- Do you no longer get pleasure from things you used to like?
- Do you often have feelings of hopelessness?

If you answered yes to any of these questions, you are likely to be depressed.

Consider how your emotional condition is affecting your life:

- Do you have a poor appetite, or do you overeat?
- Do you not sleep enough, or do you sleep too much?
- Do you have low energy or fatigue?
- Do you feel bad about yourself in general?
- Do you have trouble concentrating or making decisions?

If you answered yes to any of these questions, you may have serious depression. Seek help from your doctor or a mental health counselor.

HOME TREATMENT

Activity is the natural antidote for depression. Regular exercise can be as effective for mild depression as the drugs prescribed by doctors.

Stay involved with other people and let them support you. Tell someone about your problems. Don't push everyone away, and don't let your depression drive them away.

Drugs can cause depression, including tranquilizers, high blood pressure medicines, corticosteroids (e.g., prednisone), codeine, and indomethacin. If you are concerned about prescription medication, talk with your doctor. Reduce your other alcohol and drug use.

WHAT TO EXPECT

The doctor will ask about issues and events related to depression. The doctor may offer suggestions for activities and exercise. He or she may adjust the dosage of medication that may be causing depression.

The doctor may prescribe antidepressant medication. You may be hospitalized if there is a risk of suicide.

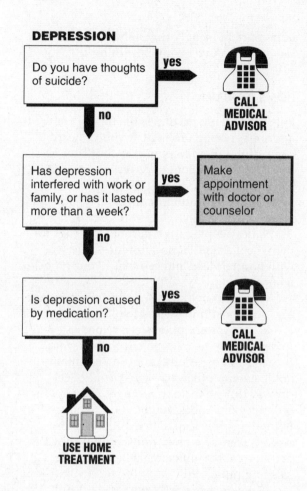

DEPRESSION

Do you have thoughts of suicide? — **yes** → **CALL MEDICAL ADVISOR**

↓ **no**

Has depression interfered with work or family, or has it lasted more than a week? — **yes** → Make appointment with doctor or counselor

↓ **no**

Is depression caused by medication? — **yes** → **CALL MEDICAL ADVISOR**

↓ **no**

USE HOME TREATMENT

SUICIDAL FEELINGS

If the depression is so severe that you are thinking of suicide, call the doctor immediately. Many communities have telephone hotlines for crisis counseling. If there is no hotline in your community, go to the nearest emergency room.

SLEEP DISORDERS

Almost everybody suffers from sleep problems now and then. Millions of people snore each night. Many people have occasional insomnia. And for 15 to 20 million Americans, sleeplessness is an ongoing problem.

Medical problems can affect the quality of your sleep. Conditions that cause pain or shortness of breath may make sleep difficult. Depression and stress can also affect sleep. In these cases, treating the underlying cause is the best way to sleep soundly again.

For many people snoring is just a noisy annoyance. However, a few snorers actually stop breathing for 30 or more seconds several times during the night. This condition, called obstructive sleep apnea, has the following signs:

- Loud, repeated snoring
- Feeling tired during the day, and taking naps

By contrast, a person with central sleep apnea produces no loud, repeated snoring, but still stops breathing briefly during sleep. The signs of this condition are:

- Waking up many times during the night, often feeling short of breath
- Seldom taking naps, though one may feel tired

Most central sleep apnea occurs in men. Doctors have linked sleep apnea with heart disease, high blood pressure, and impotence in men. Fortunately, doctors offer a range of effective treatments for it.

HOME TREATMENT

Often a sleeping partner is the first to know of a serious snoring problem. If you've heard complaints, avoid sleeping on your back, which allows the tongue to rest against the back of the throat. Losing weight is one of the least expensive and most effective treatments for snoring.

Many people turn to alcohol or drugs to help them sleep. These substances interfere with normal sleep and can make your problems worse.

While alcohol has a sedating effect, it can also act as a stimulant and may keep you awake. Nonprescription sleep remedies seem to depend on the placebo effect: they work because you expect them to. Some contain antihistamines that may cause you to feel drowsy during the day. Stronger prescription sedatives can knock you out but do not give a normal, restful sleep. Often sleeping pills make insomnia worse. You should deal with possible causes of insomnia before trying sleeping pills.

Here are some tips for a good, restful night's sleep:

- Stop smoking. Smokers have more sleep trouble than nonsmokers.
- Exercise regularly, but not in the last two hours before going to bed.
- Avoid drinking alcohol in the evening.
- Avoid caffeine for at least two hours before bedtime—coffee, tea, sodas, and chocolate.
- A bedtime snack seems to help many people, as does the traditional glass of warm milk. But don't eat a big meal within three hours of going to bed.

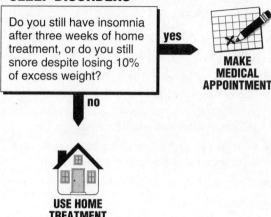

SLEEP DISORDERS

Do you still have insomnia after three weeks of home treatment, or do you still snore despite losing 10% of excess weight?

yes → **MAKE MEDICAL APPOINTMENT**

no ↓ **USE HOME TREATMENT**

- Develop a sleeping routine with a regular bedtime, but don't go to bed if you feel wide awake.
- Break your chain of thought before going to bed; read, watch television, take a bath, or listen to music to relax your mind.
- Once in bed, use creative imagery and relaxation techniques to keep your mind free of distracting thoughts.
- If all else fails (or even if it doesn't), sex is one of the most effective natural sleep inducers.

It may take you several weeks to establish a normal sleep routine. Talk to your doctor if you still have sleep problems after trying these methods.

WHAT TO EXPECT

The doctor will ask about your sleeping schedule, sources of stress and anxiety, and other sleep factors. In some cases you may have brain activity monitored (electroencephalogram, or EEG) as you sleep. Rarely, the doctor may have more sophisticated tests done during a sleep study at the hospital (polysomnography).

In rare cases where weight loss and home treatment don't stop snoring, the doctor may discuss surgery of the nose and throat.

SUBSTANCE ABUSE

Alcohol and drugs can harm every part of your life. Drinking affects your medical care in a wide range of ways, from causing certain illnesses to influencing how you react to anesthetics or pain relievers. A pregnant woman who drinks risks harming the fetus in her womb. Up to half of all domestic violence relates to substance abuse.

Five to 13% of U.S. adults abuse some kind of drug other than alcohol. Drug users risk overdose, dependency, and withdrawal symptoms. Drug users have a greater risk of disease and injury. More than one-third of all suicides are drug-related.

Because alcohol and drugs are so addictive, it is often difficult for the person with a drinking or drug problem to acknowledge needing help. A family member, a friend, or a colleague often has to take the first step. Start by seeking information from self-help groups, counselors, and your doctor.

Signs of problem drinking include:

- Drinking to get drunk
- Trying to solve or avoid problems by drinking
- Becoming loud, angry, or violent after drinking
- Drinking at inappropriate times, such as in the morning, before driving, or before going to work
- Causing problems, harm, or concern to others because of one's drinking
- Developing an ulcer or gastritis

Signs of alcoholism—medical addiction to alcohol—include:

- Spending time thinking about drinking, or planning where and when to drink
- Hiding bottles for quick pick-me-ups
- Receiving citations for driving while intoxicated, or having an automobile accident after any alcohol intake
- Starting to drink without planning to, and losing track of how much one drinks
- Denying how much alcohol one consumes
- Drinking alone
- Needing a drink before stressful situations
- Blackouts or memory loss of what occurred while drinking
- Malnutrition and neglect
- Suffering from withdrawal symptoms, including delirium tremens (DTs)

Diagnosing and treating a drug problem is even more challenging. Seek out professional help for the person who may be addicted. Don't let yourself be drawn into denying, rationalizing, or covering up the problem.

HOME TREATMENT

To find help, start by looking in your phone book under Alcohol or Drug abuse. Hotlines serve many communities around the clock. These national organizations will have local chapters in your community:

- Alcoholics Anonymous (AA)
  General Service Office
  (212) 870-3400
  www.aa.org
- Al-Anon and Alateen
  Family Group Headquarters
  (212) 302-7240
  www.alanon.alateen.org

SUBSTANCE ABUSE

If alcohol may be the problem, does the person exhibit 2 or more of these signs?

- Mentioned a need to cut down on drinking
- Acted annoyed when someone mentioned his or her drinking
- Expressed guilt about drinking
- Has taken an "eye-opener" first thing in the morning

yes → The odds are overwhelming that the person is alcoholic. Make appointment with doctor or counselor.

no ↓

Has the person displayed *any* of the above signs?

yes → This person may have a drinking problem. Discuss how it has affected your relationship.

no ↓

If drugs may be the problem, does the person exhibit any of these signs?

- Unhealthy lifestyle, neglected appearance
- Secretive behavior
- Frequent lateness or absence
- Mood swings
- Weight loss
- Money problems
- Anxiety, nervousness
- Impulsive behavior
- Troubled relationships
- Denial that the problem exists

yes → Make appointment with doctor or counselor.

no ↓

Consider other problems.

- National Council on Alcoholism and Drug Dependence (800) 622-2255
- National Clearinghouse for Alcohol and Drug Information (800) 729-6686 www.health.org
- Narcotics Anonymous (NA) World Service Office (818) 773-9999 www.wsoinc.com
- Nar-Anon Family Group Headquarters (310) 547-5800
- National Institute of Drug Abuse Hotline (800) 662-HELP
- Cocaine Hotline (800) COCAINE www.drughelp.org

WHAT TO EXPECT

Your doctor may suggest counseling. Hospitalization is reserved for those who need detoxification, who may go into withdrawal, or who suffer from severe mental illness. The average stay for these patients is 12 days.

There is no cure for alcoholism or substance dependence, but these conditions can be controlled. About 50 to 70% of substance abusers can achieve successful rehabilitation and recovery with good medical programs and long-term reinforcement.

VAGINAL DISCHARGE

Normal vaginal secretions are thin, clear, and painless. Abnormal vaginal discharge is common, however, and can have many causes.

Hormone changes can cause vaginal dryness and irritation in older women. You may need a prescription cream if the symptoms bother you. Forgotten tampons and other foreign bodies can cause vaginal irritation and discharge. Abdominal pain and bleeding between periods (p. 122) suggest the possibility of a serious problem.

Bacteria, viruses, and other microbes can infect the vagina and cause discharge:

- A mixture of bacteria may be responsible (nonspecific vaginitis)
- A yeast infection (monilia) can cause a white, cheesy discharge
- Trichomonas, a common microbe, can cause intense itch and a white, frothy discharge

These infections aren't serious but they are bothersome. Often the infection will go away by itself. Make an appointment with the doctor if the discharge lasts more than a few weeks.

See the doctor if it's possible someone has exposed you to a sexually transmitted disease (STD). Don't feel ashamed. Doctors treat STDs all the time. You'll be asked to name your sexual contacts. Be frank about naming people with whom you had contact—for their benefit. Information is kept strictly confidential.

Other signs to seek medical care are if:

- The discharge is more than slight
- The discharge is cheesy, smelly, or bloody
- The affected area hurts or itches
- The discharge lasts more than two weeks
- A girl with vaginal discharge has not reached puberty

HOME TREATMENT

Patience and good hygiene are the home treatment of vaginal discharge.

Douche daily with a Betadine solution (two tablespoons to a quart of water, or 30 ml to a liter) or baking soda (one teaspoon to a quart, or 5 ml to a liter). Also douche after intercourse.

Nonprescription anti-yeast creams, such as Monistat, may help you.

Call your doctor if you are taking an antibiotic such as tetracycline for some other condition. Your doctor may change the medication.

See the doctor if symptoms get worse or persist after two weeks of home treatment. Do not douche for 24 hours before your doctor's appointment.

WHAT TO EXPECT

The doctor will do a pelvic examination. He or she may obtain a culture from the vagina for laboratory analysis.

Suppositories or creams are the usual treatment of vaginal discharge. The doctor may prescribe oral medication for severe cases of fungus or trichomonas infection. If sexually transmitted disease is possible, the doctor will prescribe an antibiotic. Your sexual partner(s) may require treatment too.

VAGINAL DISCHARGE

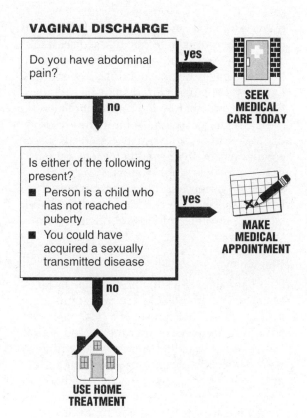

Do you have abdominal pain?

yes → **SEEK MEDICAL CARE TODAY**

no ↓

Is either of the following present?
- Person is a child who has not reached puberty
- You could have acquired a sexually transmitted disease

yes → **MAKE MEDICAL APPOINTMENT**

no ↓

USE HOME TREATMENT

MENSTRUAL PROBLEMS

The menstrual cycle varies from woman to woman. Periods may be regular or irregular, light or heavy, painful or pain-free, long or short, and yet be normal.

The rhythm of a menstrual cycle is less important than unusual changes—bleeding, pain, or discharge between periods. Menstrual problems are common. Often you can help control them with home treatment. See the doctor for problems that are severe or come back several months in a row.

Bleeding Between Periods

Many women have bleeding or spotting between menstrual periods. Women with an intrauterine birth control device (IUD) are particularly likely to have spotting. You can ignore bleeding if it is light and occasional. See the doctor if bleeding is severe or happens three months in a row. An abnormal pregnancy, cancer, or benign tumors of the uterus (fibroids) can cause such bleeding. A doctor should also evaluate any bleeding after menopause.

Difficult Periods

Mood changes and fluid retention are very common in the days just before a menstrual period. Such problems can be difficult, but they are a result of normal hormone changes during the menstrual cycle. See the doctor if problems persist for several months.

Missed Periods

There are many reasons for a late period other than the obvious one: pregnancy. Strenuous exercise, anxiety, and stress may cause missed or irregular periods. In rare cases, diseases such as hyperthyroidism upset the body's hormone balance and cause missed periods. During menopause periods may be irregular for a long time before they stop completely.

Extremes of weight—obesity or excessive dieting—can cause irregular periods. If these conditions are severe and persistent, periods may completely stop. Women who are undergoing rigorous athletic training often have irregular periods. This is rarely harmful, although it can lead to loss of calcium from the bones.

Pregnancy

Home pregnancy testing has become faster, easier, and more reliable. Home test kits are now available that can show a positive result as early as two weeks after the missed period. More sophisticated tests are available from your doctor or a laboratory. A positive result is more likely to be right than a negative one. Therefore, believe a positive test, but don't trust a negative test until you repeat it.

HOME TREATMENT

Use pads or tampons for bleeding between periods. Avoid taking aspirin, ibuprofen, naproxen, or ketoprofen—use acetaminophen for pain relief (p. 149).

Lowering salt in your diet may reduce swelling and fluid retention during the menstrual cycle. Water pills (diuretics) or hormones are rarely needed. You can take ibuprofen (e.g., Advil, Nuprin, Motrin), naproxen (e.g., Naprosyn, Aleve), or aspirin for menstrual cramps (p. 150). Products formulated for menstrual cramps (e.g., Midol) are also available.

If you miss periods, consider possible causes. If obesity may be the cause, you can

MENSTRUAL PROBLEMS

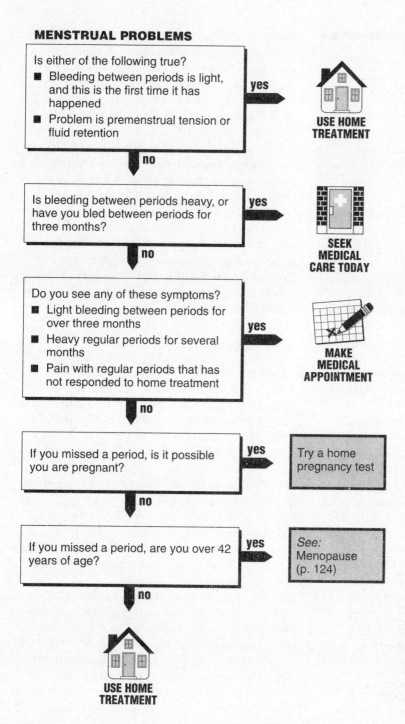

Is either of the following true?
- Bleeding between periods is light, and this is the first time it has happened
- Problem is premenstrual tension or fluid retention

yes → **USE HOME TREATMENT**

no ↓

Is bleeding between periods heavy, or have you bled between periods for three months?

yes → **SEEK MEDICAL CARE TODAY**

no ↓

Do you see any of these symptoms?
- Light bleeding between periods for over three months
- Heavy regular periods for several months
- Pain with regular periods that has not responded to home treatment

yes → **MAKE MEDICAL APPOINTMENT**

no ↓

If you missed a period, is it possible you are pregnant?

yes → Try a home pregnancy test

no ↓

If you missed a period, are you over 42 years of age?

yes → *See:* Menopause (p. 124)

no ↓

USE HOME TREATMENT

start to lose weight. If you are dieting to the point of starvation (anorexia nervosa), consult a doctor or psychotherapist. Be aware of the effects of strenuous physical exercise. If the missed periods may be due to emotional stress, identify and resolve the problem. Call the doctor if you still have questions or need help making a plan.

WHAT TO EXPECT

The doctor will do a physical examination, possibly including a pelvic exam and a Pap smear. If you have heavy bleeding, the doctor may do a dilatation and curettage (D and C). He or she may suggest other surgery depending on your diagnosis.

If you have difficult menstruation the doctor may prescribe diuretic, hormone, or some other medication. He or she may suggest therapy similar to what we describe in home treatment.

Because missed periods are rarely due to a serious medical disease, doctors rarely do a lot of tests and procedures. Doctors usually make diagnoses with a careful history and a thorough physical examination. The doctor may suggest you try a home pregnancy test.

MENOPAUSE

Many women expect that menopause will be a time of difficulty and unhappiness. Understanding the changes that take place during menopause—and what you can do about them—is the best way to approach this time of your life. You may even find that, on balance, menopause is a positive experience.

During menopause, the ovaries reduce their production of female hormones (estrogen and progesterone). Menstrual periods usually become lighter and irregular, and then stop altogether. The halt of menstrual periods means the end of fertility. After menopause a woman no longer needs contraception to prevent pregnancy. This is one aspect of menopause that many women consider positive.

Hot flashes—sudden feelings of intense heat lasting two or three minutes—are an annoying sign of menopause. They can happen anytime during the day but are most common in the evening. Caffeine and alcohol may make hot flashes worse. Exercise may improve them. For most women, hot flashes gradually decrease over about two years, and eventually disappear altogether.

Many women also have mood swings during menopause. It isn't clear whether menopausal hormonal changes cause the mood swings. The moods many women report aren't necessarily unpleasant, just unexpected. For example, one may feel alert in the middle of the night, but not uncomfortable.

Menopausal changes may also prompt a woman to worry, which is why it's good to know what changes are common. A woman in menopause may be depressed, but menopause does not cause depression.

Female hormones are responsible for the production of natural lubricants in the vagina. Loss of estrogen can cause vaginal dryness. This may lead to irritation, itching, and soreness during and after intercourse.

Osteoporosis, a condition that makes bones more fragile, begins with menopause but causes no symptoms for years. Usually the first sign of osteoporosis is a broken bone, often a hip, later in life. Such fractures are especially serious because they may lead to prolonged physical inactivity. Also, once bones become thin enough to fracture easily, it is difficult to reverse the process and strengthen the bones.

HOME TREATMENT

Staying cool is the key to treating hot flashes. Keep the home or office cool, dress lightly, and drink plenty of water. Reduce your consumption of alcohol and caffeine, and maintain a regular exercise program. There's no need for medicines such as acetaminophen or aspirin.

You can get relief from vaginal dryness with lubricants such as water-based gels (e.g., Lubifax, K-Y), unscented creams (e.g., Albolene), or other over-the-counter products (e.g., Lubrin). Many women also find that the soreness of intercourse decreases with regular sexual activity.

Regular exercise and adequate dietary calcium are important to prevent osteoporosis. An aerobic exercise program—30 minutes a day, four days a week—is good, but any physical activity will help keep bones strong (p. 131). Calcium is essential to maintain strong bones. Postmenopausal women should have 1,200 to 1,500 mg of calcium per day,

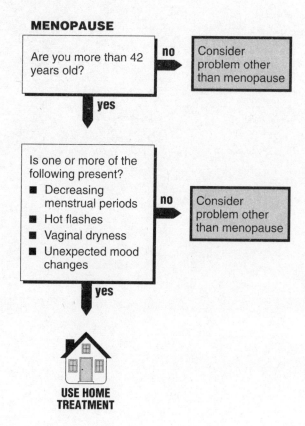

MENOPAUSE

Are you more than 42 years old? — **no** → Consider problem other than menopause

yes ↓

Is one or more of the following present?
- Decreasing menstrual periods
- Hot flashes
- Vaginal dryness
- Unexpected mood changes

no → Consider problem other than menopause

yes ↓

USE HOME TREATMENT

about as much as in a quart (1 L) of skim milk. You can use a calcium supplement if you can't get enough from dairy products.

WHAT TO EXPECT

The doctor will take the history and do a physical examination to confirm menopause.

The major issue you should discuss with the doctor is whether to take estrogen replacement therapy. Estrogen can reduce many symptoms of menopause. It also reduces the risk of heart disease, which is statistically the biggest effect. It may slightly increase your risk of uterine cancer.

Your doctor may prescribe estrogen combined with progestin, a hormone similar to progesterone. This combination may eliminate the increased uterine cancer risk and may even help protect against breast cancer. However, this combination may increase the risk of high blood pressure, heart disease, and stroke. Many doctors prescribe estrogen skin patches, which have a low dose and few side effects. However, some estrogen patches are not strong enough to strengthen the bones.

For vaginal dryness the doctor may prescribe estrogen-containing creams or suppositories. These work well and cause few side effects.

Talk over the risks and benefits of estrogen replacement therapy with your doctor.

SEXUALLY TRANSMITTED DISEASES

There are many types of sexually transmitted diseases (STDs). Their symptoms range from annoying to deadly. Fortunately, there are now treatments for all of them. Furthermore, it is important for you to know if you have an STD and may thus infect your sexual partner. For these reasons, you must not let embarrassment block you from seeking medical care.

The table below lists the symptoms of six STDs. If you think you might have any of these, you need the help of a doctor. On page 128 you'll find information about genital herpes, the only type of STD you might be able to treat at home.

Sexually Transmitted Diseases

Disease	Symptoms	Diagnosis	Treatment	Special Concerns
Gonorrhea	MEN: discharge from penis; burning feeling while urinating WOMEN: usually none; sometimes vaginal discharge and abdominal discomfort	■ Culture of a suspected infection ■ Examination of vaginal discharge by microscope	Antibiotics	Untreated can lead to: ■ Severe pelvic inflammation in women ■ Infertility ■ Arthritis ■ Other problems
Syphilis	FIRST SIGN: chancre sore in genital, anal, or mouth area LATER: rash, slight fever, swollen joints	■ Examination of fluid from chancre ■ Blood test	Penicillin or other antibiotics	Untreated can lead to: ■ Blindness ■ Brain damage ■ Heart disease ■ Birth defects
Chlamydia	Similar to gonorrhea, if any	■ Culture of a suspected infection ■ Examination of vaginal discharge by microscope	Antibiotics	Untreated can lead to: ■ Pelvic inflammation ■ Infertility in women ■ Pregnancy complications
Genital warts	Small, fleshy "condyloma" growths in genital or anal area: soft and reddish inside the body, darker growths outside	■ Physical examination	Large growths may be removed surgically or burned off	Can return after treatment
Pubic lice	■ Itching worse at night ■ Lice visible in pubic hair ■ Eggs ("nits") attached to pubic hair	■ Physical examination	Medication to kill the lice	None
AIDS (acquired immunodeficiency syndrome)	■ Unusual susceptibility to illness ■ Persistent fatigue and fever ■ Night sweats ■ Unexplained weight loss ■ Swollen glands ■ Persistent diarrhea ■ Dry cough	■ Blood test for antibodies to the human immunodeficiency virus (HIV)	Treatment can now help fight the virus and slow the disease, but there is still no cure.	Symptoms may not appear until years after infection. See page 130 for more information.

GENITAL HERPES

About 20 million Americans are infected with one of the two types of herpes virus.

- Herpes type 1 is usually spread by kissing. It causes the common fever blisters and cold sores of the lips and mouth, but can also affect the genitalia.

- Herpes type 2 usually causes infections of the genitals. It typically spreads by sexual contact, and is thus rare in children.

About one-third of those infected with herpes have bouts of red, painful blisters that last five to ten days. Illnesses, trauma, or emotional stress may trigger these episodes.

Herpes is most contagious during and just before the time when the blisters appear. Many infected people have an itchy or tingly feeling (prodrome) a day or two before the outbreak of blisters. To lower the chance of infecting someone else, avoid sexual contact when the prodrome or blisters are present. Condoms help but don't give complete protection.

Herpes infections are associated with cancer of the cervix. Therefore, if a woman has recurrent herpes infections, she has another reason to obtain a regular Pap smear test.

HOME TREATMENT

The herpes sores heal on their own, and you can't do much for them. People with fever blisters try salves, calamine lotion, alcohol, and ether. Some people may get relief, but no remedy works well. A hot bath for five to ten minutes seems to speed healing. Over-the-counter products (e.g., Blistex) may provide some relief. Many people believe that reducing stress and anxiety is helpful.

Call the doctor if the problem lasts for more than two weeks or if you're unsure your condition is herpes.

To locate a local support program, contact:

- American Social Health Association
  P.O. Box 13827
  Research Triangle Park, NC 27709
  (800) 230-6039
  www.ashastd.org

WHAT TO EXPECT

The doctor will take the history and do a physical examination. He or she will ask about your sexual habits and other personal information. It is important that you be complete and accurate.

If you have herpes, the doctor may take a sample for laboratory analysis. There are no drugs to cure herpes, but acyclovir (Zovirax) in oral form or in an ointment may make your first attack heal sooner: in 10 to 12 days rather than 14 to 16 days. The ointment usually doesn't work as well on repeated attacks. Oral acyclovir does decrease the number and severity of recurrences if you take the drug continuously, but its side effects can include nausea, vomiting, diarrhea, dizziness, joint pain, rash, and fever.

GENITAL HERPES

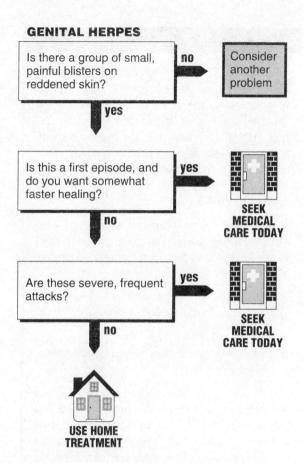

Is there a group of small, painful blisters on reddened skin?

no → Consider another problem

yes ↓

Is this a first episode, and do you want somewhat faster healing?

yes → **SEEK MEDICAL CARE TODAY**

no ↓

Are these severe, frequent attacks?

yes → **SEEK MEDICAL CARE TODAY**

no ↓

USE HOME TREATMENT

AIDS

HIV, the virus that causes AIDS, is spread primarily by:

- Sexual intercourse in which people exchange semen and vaginal fluids
- Sharing an unsterilized needle or syringe for drugs or tattoos
- Being passed from a pregnant mother to her unborn child

Doctors have not found HIV spread by saliva, sweat, tears, urine, or feces. You won't get AIDS from casual contact, such as working with someone with AIDS. Laboratories now screen the blood supply, so the risk of getting HIV from transfusions or blood products is very small.

Though AIDS is predominant in certain groups, it's not who you are but *what you do* that increases your risks. Especially risky behaviors include:

- Having multiple sex partners
- Sharing needles or syringes for drugs or tattoos
- Anal sex, with or without a condom
- Vaginal or oral sex with someone who uses IV drugs or engages in anal sex
- Sex with a stranger (pickup or prostitute), or with someone known to have multiple sex partners
- Unprotected vaginal sex with somebody who could be infected with HIV

HIV testing   Have an HIV test every three to six months while engaging in these risky behaviors, or while having sex with anyone who does. The test detects antibodies to HIV, but not the virus itself; the virus can be in your blood for months before it causes a positive test result. If the first test does detect HIV antibodies, ask for more accurate follow-up tests. It's important that you have a counselor to explain the implications of your test result and how to reduce the spread of HIV.

Prevention   Your primary means of preventing the spread of AIDS (and other STDs) is avoiding the risky behaviors listed above, and:

- Abstinence or celibacy—not having sex
- A monogamous relationship with an uninfected person
- Practicing safer sex when infection is possible

Using a latex condom reduces your risk, but a condom is not complete protection; it can break during sex. Use a water-based lubricant (e.g., K-Y), but not petroleum jelly, cold cream, or baby oil—these weaken latex. A spermicide containing nonoxynol-9 can give more protection from HIV.

Treatment   Doctors now consider AIDS a chronic disease that can be managed with medication. An expensive combination of drugs can fight the virus and bolster the immune system, but there is still no cure. There is no HIV vaccine on the horizon, and there may never be. Your best ways to prevent AIDS are avoiding risky behavior and practicing safer sex.

The Seven Keys to Health

You can do much more than any doctor or health insurer to maintain your health and well-being. The major health problems in the U.S. are severe injuries and chronic illness, such as heart disease, cancer, emphysema, and liver cirrhosis. A good plan for health can greatly reduce your risk of contracting these diseases. If you already have a disease, not only can a good health plan slow its progress, but often you can reverse some of the damage.

Your plan for good health can also prevent many nagging nonfatal health problems, such as hernias, back pain, varicose veins, and osteoporosis. By developing the habit of health, you can reduce the amount of illness you'll face in your life. You'll feel much better and have more energy. Good health is its own reward.

There are seven main ingredients in a plan for good health:

- Exercise
- Diet
- Not smoking
- Alcohol moderation
- Weight control
- Avoiding injury
- Professional prevention (i.e., medical care)

Most likely, you already take some good health measures and don't need to worry about all seven areas. You're probably already a nonsmoker. Your alcohol intake may already be moderate. Your body weight may be close to where it needs to be. So devising your plan for good health is just a matter of making improvements in areas where you've been lax.

EXERCISE

Exercise is the central ingredient in good health. It tones muscle, strengthens bone, and makes your heart and lungs work better. Exercise helps prevent heart disease, high blood pressure, stroke, and many other diseases. A sensible exercise program will increase your endurance, improve your digestion, help you sleep better at night, and enhance your overall sense of well-being.

There are three basic kinds of exercise, each with its own benefits and limitations.

- **Strengthening exercise** Traditional body-building activities—weight lifting, push-ups, or pull-ups, for example—strengthen bone and muscle, even at advanced ages. Strengthening exercise is very helpful to improve function in a body part when you need to, such as after knee surgery.

- **Stretching exercise** These exercises help keep you loose. Stretching before physical activity warms up and loosens the muscles, reducing your risk of injury. You should stretch slowly and gently, to the point of discomfort and just a little beyond. Stretching is helpful for any condition that causes joint stiffness. Do stretching exercises twice a day for any joint that can't be completely bent or straightened.

- **Aerobic exercise** This is the most important kind of exercise, the key to fitness and vitality. During aerobic exercise your body needs extra oxygen. You breathe more deeply than usual, and your lungs must work harder to process the extra oxygen you breathe in. Your heart beats faster to deliver more blood, which carries the oxygen, to your muscles. This process increases your endurance and improves the function of every cell in your body. Your lungs become able to process more air with less effort. Your heart gets larger and stronger as you get physically fit, and pumps more efficiently. As a result, your resting heart rate will be lower. And aerobic exercise burns up calories, which helps you control your weight. For aerobic exercise to be effective, you must sustain activity over time. Even 20 minutes of exercise three times a week will help. Exercising for 20 to 30 minutes five to seven days a week is ideal.

Your Activity Program

It's never too late to start an exercise program and enjoy the benefits of fitness. If you're out of shape, start at a low level and increase your effort as you gain strength and endurance.

Here are some points to keep in mind:

- A wide range of activities are good physical exercise. Jogging, swimming, and brisk walking are appropriate for all ages. A stationary bicycle or cross-country ski machine is good at home. Whatever the activity, it is important that you gradually increase the effort and duration of the exercise. Walking slowly isn't an aerobic exercise, but it's a good place to start. Gradually increase your walking up to 100 to 200 minutes per week, then move on to more strenuous exercise. Walking briskly or uphill can be aerobic if you push the pace to break a sweat and get your heart rate up. If you can't talk to a companion while you're exercising, you're probably working too hard.

- Talk to a health professional if you have a medical condition that limits your choice of exercise (especially a condition involving the heart or the joints) or if you're over age 70. Some doctors recommend that you have an electrocardiogram (EKG) before you start exercising, particularly if you're over 50 years old. We don't think these tests are necessary unless you have specific, known problems.

- Crash exercise programs are a bad idea. Start gently and go slowly. Pushing yourself too much will make you sore and want to stop. It also increases your risk of injury.

- Set goals for the level of fitness you want to achieve. Choose an aerobic activity and make it part of your daily routine. We like to see people exercise regularly at least five days a week.

- Loosen up with stretching exercises before and after your exercise. Wear clothing warm enough to keep your muscles from getting cold and cramping.

- As your training progresses, count your resting pulse rate in bed before you get up in the morning. Your goal is a resting heart rate of about 60 beats per minute. A person who is not fit may have a resting heart rate of 75 or more. Some heart specialists say that during exercise you should try to reach a heart rate equal to 220 minus your age times three-quarters. Don't worry too much about achieving a specific rate, however. There are no scientific data to justify any target heart rates.

- No exercise program comes without interruptions and problems. Common sense is the key to handling setbacks. When you begin exercising again, don't start at your previous level of activity. The general rule is to take as long to get back to your old level of activity as you were inactive. If you didn't exercise for two weeks, gradually increase your activity over a two-week period to get back to your previous level.

- Exercise should be fun. Often it doesn't seem so at first, but after you make exercise a habit you'll wonder how you ever got along without it. Once you're fit you can take advantage of your body's increased strength and stamina. You'll feel better, look better, and be healthier.

DIET

Diet is a major factor for a healthy life. Develop good dietary habits slowly over time. Here are the most important things for Americans to look out for:

- Too much saturated fat is the worst problem in the typical American diet. The U.S. government's *Healthy People 2000* goals call for people to reduce their total fat intake to less than 30% of the total calories they consume, and their saturated fat intake to less than 10%. We suggest you try to take in only 7% of your total calories as saturated fat. Here are some suggestions for removing saturated fat from your diet:

    - Cook with *natural* monosaturated fat (e.g., olive oil) or polyunsaturated fat (e.g., corn oil, soft margarine) rather than saturated fat (e.g., butter).

- Use low-fat or nonfat milk instead of whole milk.
- Avoid animal fats. Chicken and other poultry usually contain less fat than red meat if you remove their skin.
- Avoid fried foods.

■ Get more of your dietary protein from grains, low-fat meats (e.g., chicken), and fish. The best fish for you are high-fat fishes that live in cold water, such as salmon and mackerel. These contain a kind of oil that is good for your heart and lowers your serum cholesterol level.

■ Substitute complex carbohydrates (e.g., whole-grain foods and cereals) for some of the fat and protein in your diet. Complex carbohydrates are digested more slowly and provide a good source of energy.

■ Reduce the salt (sodium) in your diet. The average person in the U.S. takes in about 12 grams of sodium each day, one of the highest levels in the world. The recommended amount of salt intake is 4 grams a day. You'll get plenty of salt in your food without adding more. People with problems of high blood pressure, heart failure, or certain other difficulties may need to reduce salt even more.

■ Eating enough fiber is important. Fiber is the indigestible residue of food that passes through the entire bowel and is then eliminated in the stool. Dietary fiber (vegetables, apples, beans, whole-grain breads and cereals) helps lower your serum cholesterol. These natural sources of fiber are much better for you than laxatives and bowel stimulants.

■ Everybody needs calcium. Women over age 50 should have at least 1,500 milligrams (mg) of calcium each day, and men over age 65 at least 1,000 mg. A glass of nonfat milk contains about 250 mg of calcium. Many people need some sort of calcium supplement. The most popular forms are Tums and Oscal; each tablet contains 500 mg of calcium. One or two tablets a day will usually do it. Weight-bearing exercise, such as walking, helps stimulate your body to absorb more calcium and to develop stronger bones.

■ Medical research suggests that aspirin (80 mg daily) is effective in preventing heart attacks and stroke. Vitamin E (400 units daily) may also be effective. There is some evidence that multivitamins containing folic acid and vitamin B_6 (pyridoxine) also help. If you are over 40, ask your doctor about these simple preventive measures.

NOT SMOKING

Cigarette smoking kills 400,000 people in the U.S. each year. It is the major cause of lung cancer and emphysema, and contributes to heart disease and stroke. Although smoking a pipe or cigar doesn't cause as much lung disease, it can lead to cancer of the lips, tongue, or esophagus. The effects of chewing tobacco and snuff are similar; *smokeless* doesn't mean *harmless*.

It's never too late to quit. People who quit smoking enjoy major health benefits for the rest of their lives. Your risk of a heart attack begins to drop within a week of quitting, and returns to average within two years. Although the lung damage of emphysema is permanent, for many people the disease stops progressing when they quit smoking. Two years after quitting, your risk of lung cancer drops up to a third, and within ten years it is nearly normal.

When you quit smoking, you'll notice rewards: better-tasting food, no more nagging cough, more energy and stamina, more money and free time, fewer holes in your clothes. If you have children you'll be a better role model. You'll also be there for their future.

Here are some tips for quitting:

- Decide firmly that you really want to quit smoking. Set a date on which you'll stop. Announce this date to your friends. When the day comes, stop.

- The withdrawal from nicotine may make you nervous and irritable for about 48 hours. After that there is no further *physical* addiction. The *psychological* craving for nicotine can last a very long time or go away quickly.

- Nicotine chewing gum and nicotine patches are available without a prescription. These can help satisfy your craving for nicotine. Follow the directions and taper off nicotine from all sources over a period of weeks.

- Write down all your reasons for wanting to stop smoking. Read this list every so often to remind yourself.

- Have plenty of carrots, celery, and sugarless gum and candy on hand to keep your hands and mouth busy.

- Reward yourself every week or so by buying a treat with what would have been cigarette money.

- Combine your stop-smoking program with an increase in exercise. The two changes fit together naturally. Exercise will take your mind off smoking and reduce the tendency to gain weight.

Most health educators think that the best way to stop smoking is all at once—cold turkey. But tapering off may work better for some people. For example, you may decide to stop smoking in public first, or have your first cigarette of the day an hour later each day. Or smoke less of each cigarette, putting it out half-way. Find out what works for you, and stick with it.

The American Cancer Society, the American Lung Association, local hospitals, and other agencies offer stop-smoking courses. Try quitting smoking on your own first. If you still need help, there's a lot of it around.

ALCOHOL MODERATION

Excessive alcohol intake is a serious problem for many people in every age group. Drinking too much leads to depression, danger, and disease. Among its potentially fatal complications are liver disease, alcohol-related injury, and delirium tremens (DTs) from alcohol withdrawal. Alcohol causes many other problems that aren't fatal but that decrease your quality of life.

Fortunately, alcoholism is a disease from which many people recover. That recovery is a lifelong process. Success depends on personal characteristics, early treatment, the quality of counselors or support program, access to the right medical services, and the strong support of family, friends, and coworkers.

Usually alcoholism gets too little attention too late. Be alert for alcohol-related problems in family and friends, express your concerns to them, and help them establish a program for alcohol control or elimination. You can save their lives, and perhaps even your own. (For more information, see page 118.)

WEIGHT CONTROL

Weight control is a difficult task. It requires your continual attention. Think of it as *fat* control and it will fit in well with your other good health habits.

Exercise is an important part of weight control. Obesity isn't just the result of overeating, but also of a lower level of activity. Weight is a balance between energy consumed and energy spent. Thirty-five hundred calories equals about one pound (450 g) of fat. If you take in 3,500 calories fewer than you burn, you lose a pound of fat. If you take in 3,500 more than you burn, you gain a pound of fat.

There are two important phases to weight control: the weight-reduction phase and the weight-maintenance phase. The weight-reduction phase is the easiest. The method you use to lose weight doesn't matter much, although you should check with your health care professional if you plan to lose a large amount of weight quickly. You want to be sure that the diet you intend to follow is sound. During weight-loss, many of the calories you use daily come from burning your own body fat and protein for fuel. You need less fat and less protein in your diet during this period.

If you set a target, tell people what you're trying to do, and stick with it for a while, you can probably lose weight. One pound a week is a reasonable goal. This requires eliminating the equivalent of one day's food each week.

The weight-maintenance phase involves staying at the desirable weight you've achieved. This is more difficult, and it requires continual attention. Weigh yourself regularly and record the weight on a chart. Draw a red line at 3 pounds (2 kg) over your desired weight and maintain your weight below the line, using whatever method works best for you. Keep exercising. Accept no excuses for gaining weight. It's easier and healthier to adjust what you eat than to counter binges of overeating with crash diets. Keep yourself off the dietary roller coaster. Failure at weight maintenance accounts for most diet failures.

AVOIDING INJURY

It seems simple, but it's important: you stay healthy by not letting yourself get hurt.

- Always wear automobile seat belts, whether you're a driver or passenger. When transporting young children, use age-appropriate safety seats, and put these in the proper place.
- Make sure children wear helmets and other appropriate safety equipment when they bicycle, skateboard, skate, and engage in sports. Watch them carefully when they jump on trampolines.
- Don't drive under the influence of drugs or alcohol. Never ride in a car with an impaired driver.
- Prevent drowning by keeping an eye on children when around water. Teach your children proper pool safety. Wear life preservers on small boats.
- Make sure your home has working smoke detectors. Check their batteries yearly.
- Prevent falls in the home by avoiding clutter, putting hand rails in the bathroom, and making sure stairs are well-lit.
- If you have guns in your house, lock ammunition securely away from the firearm.

PROFESSIONAL PREVENTION

The most important part of prevention—developing good health habits—is your personal responsibility. You sometimes need professional advice as well. Preventive medicine includes five strategies that involve health professionals:

- The checkup or periodic health examination
- Screening to detect problems early
- Early treatment for problems

- Immunizations and other public health measures
- Health risk assessment

The next section has more advice on working with your health care team.

According to an old joke, everything pleasurable is either illegal, immoral, or fattening. In fact, exactly the opposite is true. Health is pleasurable, and ill health is miserable. Exercise makes you feel better. A good diet makes you feel better. Not smoking makes you feel better. Having a good body weight makes your activities easier and more pleasurable. People with good health habits develop signs of aging about eight years later than those with poor health habits. Good health habits bring along their own rewards.

Your Health Care Partners

Maintaining good health involves a partnership between you and your health care team: your doctor, your nurses, and other health professionals; and your health plan. It is important that you and your team communicate well—talking and listening to each other—so that you can make smart decisions.

You should have one personal doctor who coordinates your medical care. At times that doctor might refer you to:

- A nurse practitioner, for day-to-day problems
- A medical specialist, to diagnose and treat less common problems
- An expert in another field, such as nutrition

Your primary care doctor will also help you to understand the procedures of your health plan so that you get the best care available.

THE MEDICAL APPOINTMENT

When you make an appointment with your doctor or nurse practitioner, your first responsibility is to show up on time, or to call the office to say that you can't. This will help your doctor's office to be more efficient for everyone.

Your next responsibility is to give your doctor a concise and organized description of your illness. The office may be set up to receive this information on a form or by computer, or your doctor or nurse may collect it by talking to you.

In a complete physical examination, a doctor gathers information in the following five categories. Depending on your illness, the doctor may not have to go into all of these areas.

Chief Complaint

The doctor may ask, "What brings you here today?" or "What's the trouble?" or "What bothers you the most?" Explain the problem as best you can. What prompted you to call the doctor? Was it a sore throat? A pain? Something else out of the ordinary? Express yourself clearly. Don't worry about medical terms.

Present Illness

Next your doctor will ask more detailed questions about your chief complaint: When did it begin? What were you doing when symptoms started? What makes symptoms better or worse? Think about these questions in advance. Tell the doctor if you're unsure of dates; answer as best you can. The doctor will then learn the sequence of events from the beginning of symptoms to the present time.

Medical History   Your doctor will ask about your general health: childhood illnesses, hospitalizations, surgery, allergies, and medications. Give direct, brief answers. Give complete information about medications you've taken before or during the illness, including birth control pills, vitamins, pain relievers, and laxatives. It may be helpful to bring medication bottles to the doctor. Tell the doctor if you're pregnant, or might be pregnant. If you have allergies, describe the kind of reaction you have.

Review of Systems   In a complete exam, your doctor will ask you about possible problems with your heart, lungs, kidneys, and other bodily systems.

Social History   Your doctor may ask about your job, family, stresses, smoking, drinking, drug use, sexual activity, even exposures to chemical or toxic substances. These questions are sometimes very personal. However, truthful and complete answers may be very important in your diagnosis and treatment.

ASKING QUESTIONS   You must completely understand your health care so that you can fully participate in it. Don't worry about making a pest of yourself by asking questions. Good health professionals encourage their patients to ask questions and to take an active role in their own health care. Make a list of your questions and concerns *before* the appointment. This will help you get the most out of your office visit. When you leave the office, you should understand all information you received in the following three areas.

Instructions   Ask questions if you aren't absolutely sure about what the doctor has advised you to do. Write down the instructions, or ask the doctor to do it for you. Do not depend on your memory. Call back if you're not sure; don't try to guess.

Drugs   If you leave the appointment with a prescription or the advice to take an over-the-counter drug, you should know the purpose of the drug, its possible side effects, and how long you need to take it. Sometimes you need to keep taking the medication until the prescription runs out; other times you should stop taking the drug once you feel well. Your pharmacist is another valuable source of drug information.

Hospitalization   If your doctor recommends that you go to a hospital for tests, surgery, or other procedures, be sure you understand why and for how long.

Review the list of questions on page 141 before your medical appointment. Make sure you leave with answers to all of the questions that apply to you.

Question List

General questions to ask:
- What is my problem?
- What does the diagnosis mean?
- Could the problem be anything else?
- How likely is that?
- What is likely to happen?
- Can you tell me what [any words you don't understand] mean?
- What are my choices for the next step?
- What are the benefits, risks, and cost of each choice?

If the doctor suggests tests:
- What will we learn from these tests?
- Will they be uncomfortable?
- Do I need to make special arrangements (not eating before the test, being driven home afterward)?

If the doctor suggests medication:
- How will the medication help?
- Does it have any side effects I should know about?
- Is it available in a generic form?
- Might it interact badly with other drugs or with foods?
- What can I expect in the next few weeks and also over the long term?
- How long should I continue taking this drug?

If the doctor suggests surgery or other medical procedures:
- What are the risks of the procedure?
- How frequently does this procedure relieve this kind of problem?
- Must the procedure be done right away? Why?
- Can this be done safely as an outpatient procedure?
- How often do you do this procedure?
- I would feel more comfortable with another opinion. Could you recommend someone for me to check with?

If the doctor suggests hospitalization:
- Can I have the tests or treatment done as an outpatient?
- What are the risks of being in the hospital?
- Which hospital do you suggest and why?
- Does the hospital staff perform this treatment frequently?
- Can I recover at home and shorten the hospital stay?
- What should I do at home?
- Is there anything I shouldn't do?
- When should I check back with you?
- Should I avoid aspirin for a week or more before the procedure?

PRESCRIPTION DRUGS

Drugs are lifesaving, and they are dangerous. They can cause pain, and they can relieve pain. They can cure you, and they can make you ill. Even when they work as intended, drugs can irritate the digestive tract, cause allergic reactions, and lead to other serious problems.

You don't want to take any medications you don't really need. Some people expect a prescription every time they visit the doctor. Otherwise they feel they haven't received their money's worth. If you don't receive a prescription, that's *good.*

Most drugs don't cure, but give partial relief of symptoms such as pain or cough. If you demand urgent relief from different symptoms every time you visit the doctor, you'll likely receive more drugs than you really need. Try home treatment before you resort to medications.

If you must take medication, take the fewest drugs for the shortest possible time. Take your medications as directed—the right amount at the right times, for as long as instructed. Expect the doctor to review your needs every time you visit.

Controlling Costs

If your doctor prescribes a brand-name drug, ask if there is a lower-cost generic drug available. In many states pharmacists are permitted to fill a prescription with the appropriate generic.

If you'll be taking medication for a long time, ask the doctor to allow refills of the prescription. This will enable you to get more medication without having to pay for another office visit. Sometimes, however, the doctor will want to see you again before continuing the medication.

Check with your health plan about what pharmaceutical arrangements it has made. Pharmacies sell identical drugs, but one store may charge you more than another. Once you have found a pharmacy with prices and service that you like, keep your business there. Having one outlet fill all your prescriptions helps prevent bad drug interactions and other problems.

Managing Medications

During your appointment, you and your doctor should arrange a daily medication schedule that's convenient and effective. If the program isn't clear to you, ask the doctor to explain it.

Make a chart of your medication dosage. Mark off when you take a dose.

If you have pills left at the end of treatment, flush them down the toilet. A medicine chest full of old prescription drugs is a health hazard.

DOING YOUR PART

It's important that you follow the therapy prescribed by your doctor. Rest if you've been told to. Do the recommended exercises. Take medication correctly. Call the doctor if you have side effects, or return to the office if necessary.

For each member of your family, keep a record of this important information:

- Blood type
- Allergies and special conditions
- Immunizations and childhood diseases
- Hospitalizations (when and why)

Update the family medical record when you return from the doctor. This information may be very important in emergencies. Take the record with you to a doctor's appointment if necessary.

IMMUNIZATIONS

Only a few years ago, smallpox, cholera, polio, diphtheria, whooping cough, and tetanus killed large numbers of people throughout the world. Immunizations (vaccinations) have controlled these diseases in the United States. Smallpox has been eradicated from the entire planet. With a chicken pox vaccine available, that disease may soon become a thing of the past as well.

Unfortunately, many Americans have become lax about childhood immunizations. As a result, measles, mumps, and rubella are on the upswing. You and your children can reap the benefits of immunizations while minimizing their risks by following the vaccination schedule below. In addition:

- Keep a record of your family's immunizations. Don't get vaccinated twice just because you lost your records.

- If you haven't had a tetanus shot for ten years or so, ask for a booster shot the next time you routinely visit your doctor.

Talk to your doctor if you have any other questions about immunizations.

Recommended Immunization Schedule

Age	Immunization
Newborn	Hepatitis B (or later, as directed by doctor)
2 months	DPT (diphtheria, pertussis, tetanus), OPV (oral polio virus), and HIB (hemophilus influenza type B)
4 months	DPT, OPV, and HIB
6 months	DPT, OPV (in some areas, not in the U.S.), and HIB
15 months	Measles, Mumps, Rubella
18 months	DPT and OPV
4–6 years	DTap (diphtheria, tetanus, acellular pertussis) and OPV
5–18 years	Measles, Mumps, Rubella
Every 10 years	T(d) (adult tetanus, diphtheria)
Over 65 or when at high risk	Influenza
Over 65 or when at high risk	Pneumococcal

Supplies to Keep on Hand

You can prepare for most minor illnesses by keeping a few remedies and supplies in your home. To save money, buy only the items you will need often, and buy the inexpensive brands. The table opposite lists the products we recommend that you keep on hand. You can do almost all the home care described in this book with these items.

This chapter discusses dosages and side effects of some common medicines. Keep these points about drugs in mind:

- Always read the manufacturer's information for every product because that information can change. Talk to your doctor or pharmacist if you have questions.

- Medications eventually go bad, so you should replace them at least every three years. Check your medicine cabinet; you may find items that have expired or that you don't need.

- Keep all drugs out of reach of children. No bottle is totally childproof.

- All drugs can cause side effects, even when you use them properly. Many common medicines have unavoidable side effects, such as drowsiness.

- Don't assume that a drug is safe just because it doesn't require a prescription. Misusing over-the-counter drugs can be dangerous.

- The drugs in this chapter may relieve symptoms, but they aren't cures. If you can get along without drugs, you're usually better off.

- For most medicines, different brands are available. Look for the one with the best price. A brand-name drug is not necessarily better than a less costly generic or off-brand drug.

Home Pharmacy

Item	Use
ESSENTIAL	
Bandages and adhesive tape	To close and protect minor wounds
Antiseptic cleanser (3% hydrogen peroxide, iodine)	To clean minor wounds
Thermometer	To measure body temperature
Pain and fever relievers (acetaminophen, aspirin, ibuprofen, naproxen, or ketoprofen)	To relieve pain and reduce fever
Antacids	To relieve upset stomach
Baking soda	To treat skin irritation and soak wounds
RECOMMENDED FOR FAMILIES WITH SMALL CHILDREN	
Syrup of ipecac	To induce vomiting in some cases of poisoning
Liquid acetaminophen	To relieve pain and fever in young children
Acetaminophen suppositories	For children who can't swallow other medicine
OPTIONAL	
Antihistamines and decongestants	For symptoms of allergies
Nose drops and sprays	For runny nose or congestion
Cold tablets	For symptoms of cold
Cough syrup	For cough
Bulk laxatives	For constipation
Diarrhea remedies	For diarrhea
"Artificial tears" eye drops	For irritated eyes
Zinc oxide	For hemorrhoids
Antifungal medication	For athlete's foot and other fungal infections
Hydrocortisone cream or ointment	For rashes
Sunscreen	To prevent sunburn
Wart removers	To remove some warts
Elastic bandages	For sprains and strains

COLD AND COUGH REMEDIES

ANTIHISTAMINES AND DECONGESTANTS

Purpose

To treat allergy symptoms. Usually these remedies contain an antihistamine and a decongestant, and sometimes acetaminophen. Examples: Actifed, Allerest, Benadryl, Chlor-Trimeton, Dimetapp, Sinarest, Sudafed.

If these drugs give you relief, you may take them for several weeks through allergy season without seeing a doctor. Since allergy medications always impair your functioning to some degree, you're better off avoiding substances that cause allergies than taking drugs.

Reading the Label

The decongestant is usually pseudoephedrine or phenylpropanolamine. The antihistamine is often chlorpheniramine, diphenhydramine, or brompheniramine.

Dosage

Take according to directions. Reduce the dose if you have side effects, or try a different remedy.

Side Effects

These are usually minor and clear up if you stop taking the drug or lower the dose. Too much decongestant can cause agitation and insomnia. Antihistamine can cause drowsiness.

NOSE DROPS AND SPRAYS

Purpose

To treat a runny nose. A decongestant is the active ingredient, often ephedrine or phenylephrine. The drug shrinks nasal tissues and reduces the secretions. Examples: Afrin, Neo-Synephrine, Sinarest, Vicks.

Nose drops and sprays have problems. The major drawback is that the relief is temporary, so you want to repeat the dose. Eventually your nose can no longer respond, producing congestion worse than before. Therefore, *use nose drops or sprays for no more than three days at a time.* After several days' rest, you may use them again for up to three more days.

Dosage

Nasal drops and sprays are usually used wrong. You must bathe the swollen nasal membranes on the inner sides of the nose. If you can taste the drug, it's reaching the wrong area. Apply small amounts of liquid to the right nostril while lying on your right side for a few minutes. Then roll onto your left side and repeat with the left nostril. Use four times a day if needed but for no more than three days at a time.

Side Effects

Prolonged use of nasal drops and sprays can result in severe congestion. If you swallow a large amount of the drug, you may have a rapid heart rate and agitation. The drug may dry nasal passages and lead to nosebleeds.

COLD TABLETS

Purpose

To relieve symptoms of colds and flu. Many of these remedies give good symptomatic relief, but we think most people with colds and flu do fine with fluids and a pain reliever. Examples: Actifed, Contac, Coricidin, Dimetapp, Triaminic, dozens of others.

These compounds usually have three basic ingredients. The most important is a fever and pain reducer: acetaminophen, aspirin, ibuprofen, or naproxen. In addition, there is a decongestant drug to shrink swollen membranes, and an antihistamine to block allergies and to treat a runny nose.

Some products combine ingredients, for a "shotgun approach" to cold symptoms. As a rule, single drugs are preferable to combinations. You can treat symptoms more selectively, while taking fewer drugs and risking fewer side effects.

Reading the Label

The decongestant is often pseudoephedrine or phenylpropanolamine. The antihistamine is often chlorpheniramine (Chlor-Trimeton, etc.) or diphenhydramine.

Scopolamine or belladonna may be added to enhance effects and reduce stomach spasms.

Don't use products with caffeine if you have heart trouble or difficulty sleeping.

The commonly prescribed cold medicines (e.g., Sudafed, Actifed, Dimetapp) are just more concentrated and expensive versions of the same drugs available over the counter—often under the same brand names.

Dosage

Try the recommended dosage. If you feel no effect you may increase the dosage by one-half. Don't exceed twice the recommended dosage. Increasing the dosage may enhance your relief of symptoms but brings a greater risk of side effects.

Side Effects

There are no common serious side effects to cold and flu medicines. The most common side effects of cold tablets are drowsiness and agitation. Drowsiness is usually caused by the antihistamine, while insomnia or agitation results from the decongestant. You can try another compound that has less of the offending drug, or reduce the dose.

Drowsiness may make it dangerous for you to drive or operate machinery. In rare cases, some drugs may cause a dry mouth, blurred vision, or inability to urinate. Side effects of aspirin include upset stomach, ringing in the ears, and bleeding from the stomach.

COUGH SYRUPS

Purpose

Cough syrups are of two major types:

- **Expectorants** thin secretions in the lungs and airway, allowing you to cough up the bad material.
- **Suppressants** dull the cough reflex, reducing coughs by half or more.

If you have a lot of mucus, you want to cough it out. Therefore, expectorants are usually preferable. Cough suppressants are best for dry, hacking coughs that prevent sleep or work.

We discourage the use of cough syrups containing antihistamine, which dries the airway and can do more harm than good.

Reading the Label

Guaifenesin (Robitussin, Benylin expectorant, Vicks, etc.), potassium iodide, and several other compounds are expectorants.

Over-the-counter cough suppressants—such as Robitussin-DM, Triaminic-DM, Vicks Formula 44, and others—often contain dextromethorphan.

The suppressant in prescription cough syrup is mostly from narcotics, such as codeine.

Many cough syrups contain a mixture of drugs and may have some cold remedy ingredients. For example, guaifenesin is available with decongestants and cough suppressants; the remedy name may have a "-PE" suffix for phenylephrine (a decongestant ingredient), or a "-DM" for dextromethorphan.

Dosage

Follow directions on the label. Adults may require up to twice the recommended dosage of dextromethorphan, but don't exceed this amount. A higher dose may produce problems, not further benefit.

Side Effects

Cough syrup may cause drowsiness. Do not drive or operate machinery.

No significant problems have been reported with guaifenesin. If you use preparations containing other drugs you may experience side effects from these other ingredients.

FOR PAIN AND FEVER

PAIN AND FEVER MEDICATIONS

Purpose

To relieve pain and lower fever. There are five major over-the-counter drugs: acetaminophen, aspirin, ibuprofen, naproxen, and ketoprofen. Each has benefits and drawbacks.

Acetaminophen is the safest, while the others can cause severe bleeding of the stomach. On the other hand, acetaminophen doesn't reduce inflammation, while the others do. Ibuprofen and naproxen are better for relieving menstrual cramps.

Pain reliever makers often conceal key drugs in the fine print under "active ingredients." It can be hard to find out what is in each product. Keep in mind that while there are many brands, there are only five drugs. Each company wants its product to appear unique, so each develops minor variations on a theme and tries to create distinctive advertising.

For example, Anacin is aspirin and caffeine (caffeine improves pain relief but may make you jittery); Anacin 3 is acetaminophen; Excedrin is half aspirin and half acetaminophen. Bufferin and Ascriptin add an antacid to reduce stomach distress. Other than these variations, there's little reason to prefer one product over another. If you prefer tablets to caplets, choose them. If you like a particular brand, use it. If you want to save money, read labels carefully and look for the best buys.

Some pain reliever bottles have U.S.P. on the label, which stands for "United States Pharmacopoeia." Although not a guarantee that the drug is superior, it does mean that the drug meets certain manufacturing standards. The same is true of the designation N.F., which stands for "National Formulary."

Remember that acetaminophen, ibuprofen, naproxen, and ketoprofen are available by doctor's prescription at up to twice the strength of the nonprescription formulas. If you have the stronger version of a drug in your medicine cabinet, don't confuse it with the weaker over-the-counter formula.

ACETAMINOPHEN

Acetaminophen is available in several brand-name products: Datril, Liquiprin, Tempra, Tylenol, and others. Acetaminophen is a good choice for adults because of its safety, and it's our first choice for children and teenagers. Acetaminophen lacks the anti-inflammatory action that makes aspirin valuable to treat arthritis and other diseases. On the other hand, it doesn't have aspirin's common side effects. Nor can it cause Reye's syndrome, a rare but serious potential side effect of aspirin when taken by children with chicken pox or the flu.

Dosage

You take acetaminophen in doses identical to those of aspirin. For adults, two 325 mg tablets every three to four hours is standard. In children, the dose is 65 mg per year of age every four hours. There's no reason to exceed these doses because there's no additional benefit in taking higher amounts. Like aspirin, acetaminophen comes combined with other ingredients in products that offer few advantages.

Side Effects

Acetaminophen rarely causes side effects. An overdose can cause life-threatening liver failure, particularly in children. Keep the bottle out of their reach. Do not take acetaminophen if you're drinking alcohol heavily; this can cause severe liver damage. Do not exceed the recommended maximum dose of 4 grams (that's 12 regular-strength tablets) per day.

LIQUID ACETAMINOPHEN FOR SMALL CHILDREN

For a small child, most pediatricians prefer liquid acetaminophen or sodium salicylate over aspirin. The liquids are easier to swallow and better tolerated by children. Call your doctor if the child is unable to keep the medication down because of vomiting. The doctor may prescribe aspirin suppositories.

Dosage

Drug companies make liquid acetaminophen in different strengths. Read the label for the correct dosage. Usually, give 65 mg of acetaminophen for every year of the child's age, every four hours. If necessary wake the child to give acetaminophen from noon to midnight. After midnight fevers usually break; if you miss a dose then, it's less important. However, check the child's temperature at least once during the night to make sure. Acetaminophen lasts only about four hours in the body. You must keep repeating the dose or you'll lose the effect.

ASPIRIN

Expensive aspirin products may use coated tablets for easier swallowing, or they may dissolve faster, but this usually doesn't make them more effective than cheaper brands.

If an aspirin bottle contains a vinegary odor when opened, the pills have begun to deteriorate. Throw them away. Aspirin usually has a shelf life of about three years.

Dosage

The standard dose for adults is two tablets every three to four hours, as needed. Aspirin takes about two hours to achieve the maximum effect.

Each standard tablet is 5 grains, or 325 mg. The terms "extra strength," "arthritis pain formula," and others usually just indicate a greater amount of aspirin per tablet. A typical extra-strength tablet may contain 400 to 500 mg of aspirin. You may save money by taking more tablets of a less expensive brand.

With aspirin, more isn't always better. You won't get more relief by increasing the dose over 650 to 1,000 mg every four hours, and you're more likely to irritate your stomach.

Don't give aspirin to children or teenagers with a fever because of the risk of Reye's syndrome, a potentially fatal disease of the liver and brain. If aspirin is all that's available, give no more than 65 mg for every year of the child's age.

Aspirin treats symptoms; it doesn't cure problems. For symptoms such as headache or muscle pain, take aspirin only when you actually feel pain. On the other hand, to control a fever, you'll be more comfortable if you repeat the dose every four hours during the day. Afternoon and evening are usually the worst for fever, so try not to miss a dose during these hours.

Aspirin is also used to prevent heart attacks and complications of high blood pressure during pregnancy. The dose in these cases is very low: one baby aspirin (81 mg) every day. Talk to your doctor before taking aspirin for these reasons.

Side Effects

Besides Reye's syndrome in children, aspirin

DOSAGES FOR CHILDREN

For children under ten, the dose of both aspirin and acetaminophen is 65 mg for each year of the child's age, given every four hours. For example, a six-year-old child should receive no more than 380 mg (65 x 6 = 380) every four hours. Once children are ten years old, they can take the adult dose.

can cause an upset stomach or ringing in the ears in adults and children. If your ears ring, reduce the dose.

Aspirin can cause serious digestive system hemorrhage or a perforated stomach. Aspirin more than doubles your risk of a bleeding ulcer. Other problems linked to aspirin include asthma, nasal polyps, and deafness.

If your stomach is upset, try taking aspirin a half-hour after meals. Coated aspirin (e.g., Ecotrin) can help protect the stomach, but some people don't digest it at all. Buffered aspirin may help protect your stomach. If you take a lot of aspirin and want a buffered preparation, we recommend one with a nonabsorbable antacid (e.g., Bufferin). For short-term use, buffers make little difference.

ASPIRIN RECTAL SUPPOSITORIES FOR SMALL CHILDREN

Aspirin rectal suppositories are usually available by prescription. Suppositories allow medicine to be absorbed through the rectum. If you have a small child, ask your doctor about them. Use these only when vomiting prevents the child from keeping medication down. Because of their side effects and the risk of Reye's syndrome, aspirin rectal suppositories are a last resort when a child has a high fever.

Dosage

You can give small children more aspirin with suppositories than with tablets—81 mg for each year of the child's age every four to six hours. After age ten, use the adult dose. Read the label carefully. Most suppositories contain 325 mg of aspirin. You may need to cut a suppository lengthwise with a knife to make a safe dosage. As you insert the suppository into the rectum, firm but gentle pressure will make the muscles relax. Be patient. With a young child you may need to gently hold the buttocks together to keep the suppository in.

Side Effects

Besides the potential side effects of aspirin listed above, aspirin suppositories can irritate the rectum and cause bleeding. Call your doctor if you need to give more than two or three doses.

IBUPROFEN

Ibuprofen (e.g., Advil, Motrin, Nuprin) is used for arthritis, pain, and fever. Ibuprofen is about as hard on the stomach as aspirin. It doesn't have as many side effects as aspirin or acetaminophen; it's almost impossible to commit suicide by overdose with ibuprofen. Ibuprofen is sometimes more expensive than the alternatives. It's the best over-the-counter product for menstrual cramps.

(Ketoprofen, a chemical relative of ibuprofen, is also available over the counter, as Orudis KT. It offers no advantage for most people and is a little harder on the stomach.)

Dosage

Ibuprofen comes in 200 mg tablets. The maximum dose is 1,200 mg (six tablets) per day. This dose is effective for minor problems. You shouldn't take more without a doctor's advice.

Side Effects

Stomach system upset is the most common problem of ibuprofen. If you have problems, stop taking the drug and call the doctor. In rare cases ibuprofen can lead to hemorrhage or perforation of the stomach. The person who is allergic to aspirin may also react to ibuprofen. Read pain medication labels carefully.

NAPROXEN

Naproxen (e.g., Aleve over the counter, Naprosyn and Anaprox by prescription) lasts longer than other pain relievers, so you need to take it only twice a day. It is effective against pain, fever, and inflammation.

Dosage

Naproxen comes in 200 mg tablets. Read the label carefully. Don't take more than three tablets in 24 hours, no more than two if you're over 65 years old.

Side Effects

Stop taking the drug and call your doctor if you have an upset digestive system.

THERMOMETER

Purpose

To measure body temperature. The best places to measure body temperature are the rectum and the mouth. Rectal temperatures are about 0.5°F (0.25°C) higher than oral (mouth) temperatures and usually reflect the body's condition more accurately. Hot or cold foods, breathing, and smoking can affect oral temperature.

Rectal thermometers are best for young children because it's hard for them to hold an oral thermometer under the tongue. Lubricants, such as Vaseline, can make inserting rectal thermometers easier. Place the child on his or her stomach and hold one hand on the buttocks to prevent movement. Insert the thermometer an inch or so (2 to 3 cm) inside the rectum. The mercury will begin to rise within seconds. Remove the thermometer when the mercury no longer rises, after a minute or two.

You can take an oral temperature with a rectal thermometer after sterilizing it for ten

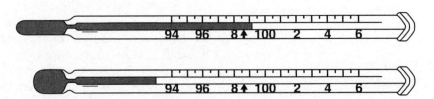

Thermometers. *Top:* Oral thermometer. Note the long, thin bulb. In this example, the mercury needs to be shaken down toward the bulb before use. *Bottom:* Rectal thermometer. The rounded bulb makes it easier to put into the rectum. This drawing shows a thermometer ready to use, its mercury shaken down.

minutes in a solution of 10 parts water to 1 part bleach. A rectal thermometer needs more time in the mouth for an accurate reading. Oral thermometers can be used to take rectal temperatures, but we don't recommend using them in children because of their shape.

Electronic thermometers, including those that take temperatures from the ear, are accurate and fast, which is useful for younger children. However, they're more expensive than mercury thermometers. Contact thermometers—strips of plastic held against the forehead—are not accurate.

Side Effects

The mercury in thermometers is poisonous. Never bite down on a thermometer.

FOR WOUNDS AND SPRAINS

ANTISEPTIC CLEANSERS

Purpose

To cleanse minor wounds. Dirt and foreign material trapped beneath the skin can lead to infection and delay healing. An antiseptic cleanser removes dirt and kills the germs. You must scrupulously clean a wound, scrubbing out any embedded dirt particles, even if it hurts and bleeds. Here are different useful cleansers:

- Plain soap and water is effective.
- A solution of 3% hydrogen peroxide is a good antiseptic. The solution foams in a wound, helping remove debris.
- Iodine is reasonably good at killing germs. Nonstinging forms (e.g., Betadine) work just as well.
- A strong baking soda solution used to soak the wound will draw out fluid and debris.

For small, clean cuts, use soap and water followed by iodine and then more soap and water. For larger wounds, use hydrogen peroxide with vigorous scrubbing.

A solution's cleansing effect is usually more important than any germ-killing activity because many products (e.g., Listerine, Zephiran, Bactine) aren't very good at killing germs. Antibiotic creams (e.g., Bacitracin, Neosporin) are expensive and usually unnecessary. First-aid sprays are a waste of money.

Dosage

Stores usually sell hydrogen peroxide as a 3% solution. Don't use a hydrogen peroxide solution stronger than 3%, such as that used for bleaching hair. Pour the 3% solution on the wound and scrub with a rough cloth. Wash and repeat until all dirt and debris are gone. Go to the doctor if you can't clean the wound.

You can paint the wound and surrounding area with iodine. Wipe it on the skin, then wash off most of it after a few minutes, leaving a trace of color on the skin.

To make a baking soda soak, mix 1 tablespoon (15 ml) in 1 cup (250 ml) of warm water. Immerse the wound if possible, or cover the wound with a washcloth soaked with the solution. Soak a wound for five to ten minutes at a time, twice a day. You can wrap the cloth compress with plastic wrap to retain heat and moisture.

Side Effects

Hydrogen peroxide is safe on skin but can bleach hair and clothing. Try not to spill it.

Iodine can irritate the skin if used full strength. Washing the area after using iodine is important. Iodine is also poisonous if swallowed; keep it away from children. Some people are allergic to iodine; stop if you get a rash.

Baking soda is completely safe if used on the skin and not swallowed.

BANDAGES AND ADHESIVE TAPE

Purpose

To close and protect minor wounds. Generally it's better to leave a minor wound open to the air than to cover it. Covering a wound can allow infection to grow beneath the bandage. Still, a home medical kit wouldn't be complete without an assortment of adhesive bandages. Bandages are useful for covering blisters, protecting a wound from dirt, and keeping the edges of a cut together.

Usage

Use an adhesive bandage for smaller cuts and sores. Leave the bandage on for a day or so. If you keep the wound covered longer, change the bandage daily.

To close a cut, apply the bandage perpendicular to the wound and draw the skin edges together. See the doctor if a wound won't stay closed or if fat is protruding from the wound.

For larger injuries, use a sterile 2 x 2 inch (5 x 5 cm) or 4 x 4 inch (10 x 10 cm) dressing, or make a dressing from a roll of gauze. Firmly secure the dressing with adhesive tape, or secure it with gauze and firmly tape this in place with adhesive tape. Change the bandage daily or if it gets wet.

Side Effects

The bandage may hide a developing infection if a wound isn't cleaned thoroughly. Some people are allergic to adhesive tape and should use nonallergenic paper tape. Adhesive tape may irritate your skin if left on for a week or so.

Some people leave a bandage on too long because they fear the pain of removing it, particularly if their hair is stuck to the tape. For painless removal, apply nail polish remover to the back of the adhesive tape and let it soak for five minutes. This will dissolve the adhesive.

ELASTIC BANDAGES

Purpose

To treat sprains and similar injuries. Elastic bandages (e.g., Ace) give gentle support to an injury and help reduce swelling. An elastic bandage is not a substitute for a splint or cast. You can reinjure yourself while wearing one. It can function best as a reminder to take it easy.

You may need a narrow or a broad elastic bandage, depending on your injury. Keep both widths on hand. One-piece supports designed for the knee, ankle, and wrist may be more convenient.

Usage

Many people think they should stretch an elastic bandage as they wrap it. That isn't necessary. Simply wrap the bandage like a roll of gauze.

Start wrapping at the far end of the injured area and work toward the trunk, making each loop a little looser as you go. For example, a knee bandage should be tighter below the knee than above.

After the discomfort is gone, keep wearing the bandage for support to allow complete healing. This usually takes about six weeks. Toward the end of the healing period, leave the bandage off except for activities likely to stress or reinjure the joint.

Side Effects

An elastic bandage can cause trouble if applied so tightly that it impairs circulation. The bandage should be firm but not tight. The limb shouldn't swell, hurt, or feel cooler beyond the bandage. Bluish or purplish skin is a sign that the bandage is too tight.

FOR SKIN CARE

ANTIFUNGAL PREPARATIONS

Purpose

To treat fungal infections of the skin. Skin fungus needs moist, undisturbed areas to grow; it will often go away with washing and drying twice a day, and powdering to keep the area dry. But if needed, effective antifungal remedies are available. For athlete's foot, try a zinc undecylenate cream or powder, such as Desenex. Tolnaftate (e.g., Tinactin) and clotrimazole (e.g., Lotrimin) are useful for difficult fungus problems.

Dosage

Use athlete's foot and jock itch remedies as directed. Selenium sulfide is effective for other skin problems. It's available by prescription, and also over the counter in a 1% solution as Selsun Blue shampoo. Apply the shampoo as a cream and let it dry on the skin. Repeat several times daily.

Side Effects

There are very few side effects from antifungal products. Too much selenium sulfide can burn the skin, so reduce if you notice any irritation. Selenium may discolor hair and will stain clothes.

Be very careful when applying any of these products around the eyes. Don't take them by mouth.

HYDROCORTISONE CREAM

Purpose

To relieve skin itching and the symptoms of skin rashes such as poison ivy and poison oak. These creams are strong anti-inflammatory products. Often they're as effective as anything your doctor can prescribe. They are safe when used for a short time. Examples: CaldeCORT, Cortizone-10, Benadryl Itch Relief Cream.

Dosage

Rub a very small amount on the rash. If you can see cream remaining on the skin, you've used too much. Repeat as often as needed, usually every two to four hours.

Side Effects

Eventually these creams can cause thinning of the skin. Limit your use to two weeks. Beyond that time, check with your doctor. These creams can make an infection worse, so be careful if a rash could be infected. Don't use these creams around the eyes, and don't take them by mouth.

SKIN CREAMS AND MOISTURIZING LOTIONS

There's little to be said about the creams, lotions, and other products that people apply to their skin in an attempt to improve its appearance or slow aging. The claims of such products are not scientifically proven.

Moisturizing creams and lotions (e.g., Lubriderm, Vaseline, Alpha-Keri) may soothe your skin and make it feel better. Use these creams as directed. They have essentially no side effects, except that some people are allergic to the lanolin in some of them.

SUNSCREENS

Purpose

To prevent sunburn. Sunscreens filter harmful ultraviolet rays, but they do not completely block out light. You can still burn, depending on the intensity of sunlight and how long you remain exposed.

The sun protection factor (SPF) number is a good guide to the blocking power of sunscreens. The higher a product's number, the better its blocking power. An SPF of 15 is good protection. For areas of the skin that are unusually sensitive to the sun, such as the nose and ears, you may need an opaque sun block such as zinc oxide.

The length of time a sunscreen stays on the skin is important. Even the best sunscreen won't help after it has washed off. Look for non-water-soluble products if you plan to be in the water.

Dosage

Apply evenly to exposed skin as directed on the label.

Side Effects

Very rarely, sunscreens can cause skin irritation and allergic reactions.

WART REMOVERS

Purpose

To remove warts. A virus causes warts. If you get one wart, you're likely to get more. Warts often go away by themselves. The exception is plantar warts, on the sole of the foot; sometimes they won't go away even with home treatment, and are painful enough to warrant a doctor's attention.

Over-the-counter remedies, such as Compound W and Wart-Off, are effective at treating warts. They contain a mild skin irritant. Repeated application slowly burns off the top layers of the wart, eventually destroying the virus.

Dosage

Apply repeatedly as directed on the product label. You must be persistent to eradicate warts.

Side Effects

Wart removers are caustic to the skin; that's how they work. Apply them only to the wart. Be very careful around your eyes or mouth.

ZINC OXIDE

Purpose

To treat hemorrhoids. Zinc oxide powders and creams soothe and protect the irritated area.

Reading the Label

Look for hemorrhoid products containing zinc oxide, such as Desitin. We discourage the use of Preparation H, Anusol, or products containing xylocaine (or other active ingredients identified by the suffix "-caine") because they can cause irritation.

Dosage

Apply as needed, following label directions. Apply after a bath when you have carefully cleaned and dried the area.

Side Effects

Essentially none.

FOR DIGESTIVE PROBLEMS

ANTACIDS

Purpose

To relieve upset stomach. There are two types of antacid, plus a new group of acid blockers that relieve heartburn in a different way:

- **Nonabsorbable antacids** help neutralize stomach acid and decrease heartburn, ulcer pain, gas pains, and stomach upset. These products are available in liquid and tablet forms. For most people, a liquid is better than tablets at coating the surface of the stomach. If carrying a bottle is cumbersome, keeping a few tablets in a shirt pocket or handbag may be easier. If not well chewed, however, tablets may be almost worthless. Examples: Amphojel, Di-Gel, Gelusil, Maalox, Mylanta.

- **Absorbable antacids** are more powerful acid neutralizers. They can cause problems down the road, however, because your stomach absorbs their active ingredients. We therefore recommend the nonabsorbable antacids, or a combination of nonabsorbable and absorbable. Most absorbable antacids come in convenient tablets. Examples: baking soda, Alka-Seltzer, Rolaids, Tums.

- **Stomach acid blockers** block the body's production of acid, rather than neutralizing stomach acid as antacids do. Tagamet (cimetidine) and Pepcid AC are acid blockers sold over the counter to treat heartburn. Most people don't need these products, but you can consider them if

antacids don't help. Check with your doctor before taking an acid blocker if you take other medications.

Different products have different tastes. Choose the brand you can stand.

Reading the Label

Nonabsorbable antacids contain magnesium and/or aluminum.

The main ingredient in absorbable antacids is sodium bicarbonate (Alka-Seltzer, baking soda), dihydroxyaluminum sodium carbonate (Rolaids), or calcium carbonate (Tums).

Dosage

The standard adult dose of antacid is 2 tablespoons (30 ml) or two well-chewed tablets. Use one-half the adult dose for children of ages six to 12, and one-fourth the adult dose for children of ages three to six.

To use baking soda, use 1 teaspoon (5 ml) in a glass of water every four hours as needed—but only occasionally.

The duration of treatment depends on the severity of your condition. One or two doses are often enough for stomach upset or heartburn. You may need several doses a day for several days for gastritis. You may need six weeks or more of treatment for an ulcer.

Side Effects

Antacids' main problem is their effect on bowel movements. Maalox (with magnesium) can cause loose stools. Amphojel and Aludrox (with aluminum) tend to result in constipation. Change brands or adjust your dose as needed.

Check with your doctor before using antacids if you have kidney disease, heart disease, or high blood pressure. People on a low-salt diet should avoid brands high in salt.

Di-Gel has the lowest salt content of the popular brands.

Baking soda is very high in sodium. Because some people should avoid sodium, we recommend using a nonabsorbable antacid instead of baking soda. Swallowing baking soda regularly for many months could also result in kidney damage.

Calcium carbonate can be mildly constipating but is a good source of supplemental calcium.

BULK LAXATIVES

Purpose

To treat constipation. We prefer a natural diet with plenty of vegetable fiber—celery, for instance—over any laxative. However, if you must use a supplement, psyllium is your best choice. Psyllium draws water into the stool, forms a gel, and provides bulk. The digestive tract does not absorb psyllium; it passes through. Psyllium is a natural product with no side effects. Examples: EfferSyllium, Metamucil, and many others.

Dosage

The typical dose of bulk laxatives is 1 teaspoon (5 ml) stirred in a glass of water, taken twice daily. Follow the laxative with a second glass of water or juice. Psyllium is also available in convenient individual-dose packets that cost more. The effervescent brands mix more rapidly and taste better to some people.

Side Effects

If you take a bulk laxative without enough water, the gel could lodge in your esophagus. Make sure you take the laxative with plenty of water or juice.

DIARRHEA REMEDIES

Purpose

To treat diarrhea. You don't need medication for occasional diarrhea. For persistent diarrhea, products with kaolin, pectin, or bismuth may help.

For "traveler's diarrhea," caused by unfamiliar bacteria, call your doctor before the trip; antibiotics such as tetracycline or doxycycline might prevent this problem.

If these remedies don't end the diarrhea, a doctor may prescribe stronger drugs such as paregoric.

Reading the Label

Diasorb, Rheaban, and similar medicines contain a mineral called attapulgite, which has a gelling effect that helps form a solid stool.

Kaopectate contains kaolin and pectin.

Pepto-Bismol and similar medications contain bismuth subsalicylate.

Dosage

Use as directed. Overall, you should treat severe diarrhea more vigorously, while minor problems require less medicine. Call the doctor for children below age three.

Side Effects

Kaolin, pectin, and attapulgite have none. Bismuth may cause a temporary, harmless darkening of the tongue and/or stool.

TO INDUCE VOMITING

SYRUP OF IPECAC

Purpose

To induce vomiting after poisoning by a plant or a drug, particularly with young children. If you have children in your home, keep syrup of ipecac on hand just in case. Vomiting will empty the stomach of poison that the victim has not absorbed. The sooner the stomach is emptied, the better off the poisoning victim will be.

Do not use syrup of ipecac or induce vomiting if:

- The person swallowed a petroleum-based compound, such as gasoline or furniture polish.
- The person swallowed a strong acid or alkali, such as drain cleaner. A poison that burns going down will burn coming up.
- The victim is unconscious. The person could inhale vomit, resulting in pneumonia.

Call the Poison Information Center immediately and follow their advice. For more information on poisoning, see page 10.

Poisoning is easier to prevent than to treat. Keep all hazardous substances out of the reach of children.

Dosage

One tablespoon (15 ml) of ipecac may be enough for a small child. Older children and adults may need 2 to 4 teaspoons (10 to 20 ml). Have the person drink as much warm water as possible until he or she vomits. Repeat the ipecac dose in 15 minutes if the person has not vomited.

Side Effects

Syrup of ipecac may cause discomfort, but it is safe. Vomiting is not hazardous unless material enters the windpipe.

VITAMIN SUPPLEMENTS

In the past, vitamin-deficiency diseases (scurvy, beriberi, etc.) were common, so there were good reasons for vitamin supplements. Today only people who are malnourished or who have conditions that interfere with absorbing natural vitamins suffer vitamin deficiency. A well-balanced diet provides enough nutrients for the average person.

On the other hand, research suggests that some kinds of vitamin supplements may be useful to prevent certain conditions. Don't expect too much: there's little evidence that vitamins will cure colds or cancer, prevent aging, or give you more energy, an enhanced immune system, or an improved sex life.

Vitamin supplements are unlikely to cause problems when taken in reasonable doses. Cheaper house brands are usually just as good as heavily advertised brands.

Here's a summary of current information on vitamin supplements:

- **Vitamin A:** may lower the risk of breast cancer among women who have had low amounts in their diet
- **Vitamin B_6:** may reduce the risk of heart disease
- **Vitamin C:** 300 mg daily may reduce risk of eye cataracts by 70%, and may reduce side effects of some cancer therapies
- **Vitamin D:** should be taken by infants who are breast-feeding
- **Vitamin E:** 400 units daily may reduce risk of heart disease by up to half, and may also reduce risk of cataracts

- **Folic acid:** 1 mg per day before and during early pregnancy greatly reduces the risk of severe nervous system defects in the child; may reduce risk of heart disease in adults

Some supplements contain many vitamins and minerals, at levels equal to or somewhat above the recommended daily allowance (RDA). One study examined a multivitamin supplement containing at least the RDA of vitamin A, beta-carotene, thiamine, riboflavin, niacin, vitamin B_6, folic acid, vitamin B_{12}, vitamin C, vitamin D, vitamin E, iron, zinc, copper, selenium, iodine, calcium, and magnesium. It found that healthy adults over age 65 who took this multivitamin reduced their number of sick days by more than half.

Dosage

Multivitamin supplements usually contain at least the RDA of each vitamin.

Side Effects

Vitamin A, vitamin D, and vitamin B_6 (pyridoxine) can cause severe problems when taken in extremely large doses. Large doses of vitamin C may cause kidney problems in rare instances. Serious side effects of other vitamins are rare.

INDEX

Boldface numbers indicate pages where you can find the most information on common medical problems. These pages usually contain decision charts and advice on home treatment and when to see a doctor.